S[E]X

IF YOU'RE SCARED OF
THE TRUTH
DON'T READ THIS!

STRAIGHT TALK FROM
A FORMER U.S. MARINE
CARL SOMMER

Medical Information Reviewed for Accuracy
by The Medical Institute for Sexual Health

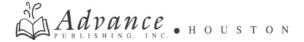

Advance . HOUSTON
PUBLISHING, INC.

Permissions
Advance Publishing, Inc.
6950 Fulton St.
Houston, TX 77022
www.advancepublishing.com
First Edition

Library of Congress Cataloging-in-Publication Data

Sommer, Carl, 1930-
Sex : if you're scared of the truth don't read this! / Carl Sommer. -- 1st ed.
    p. cm.
Includes bibliographical references and index.
ISBN-13: 978-1-57537-356-0 (library binding : alk. paper)
ISBN-10: 1-57537-356-4 (library binding : alk. paper)
ISBN-13: 978-1-57537-357-7 (pbk. : alk. paper)
ISBN-10: 1-57537-357-2 (pbk. : alk. paper) 1. Sex instruction for teenagers. 2. Teenagers--Sexual behavior. I.
Title.

HQ35.S54 2009
613.9'51--dc22

                    2008051213

Contents

Dedication

This book is dedicated to the thousands of children who have read my story books promoting principles for successful living and are now today's youth.

About the Author

Carl Sommer, a devoted educator and successful businessman, has a passion for communicating values and practical learning skills. As a successful businessman and educator, Sommer is eminently qualified to impart to students the principles necessary for success in an increasingly complex world.

Following his passion, Sommer has authored books in many categories. His works include: *Another Sommer-Time Story*™ series of children's books, read-alongs, and videos that impart values and principles for success for children; literacy programs dealing with reading; technical books, and a video math program from addition to trigonometry (see www.advancepublishing.com for the latest information about these programs).

During the Korean War, Sommer served in the Marine Corps. At age 40, he became a New York City public high school teacher. To become certified, he attended Oswego State University, City College of New York, and New York University. Sommer then became an assistant dean of boys in a high school with 3,600 pupils where he counseled students and parents.

As Sommer taught, he witnessed firsthand the many deficiencies of the educational system and began to investigate. His research led him to work as a substitute teacher at every grade level in 27 different schools in all of the boroughs of New York City. After identifying the problems and needs of America's students, he proceeded to craft solutions. His exhaustive ten-year study, including a one-year leave of absence from teaching, led to his first book published in 1984, *Schools in Crisis: Training for Success or Failure?*

Across the nation, Sommer appeared on radio and television programs, including the nationally syndicated Oprah Winfrey Show. He has served on the Texas State Board of Education Review Committee and taught a Junior Achievement economics course at Prague University, Czech Republic. The International Biographical Centre in Cambridge, England, has nominated him for International Writer of the Year.

Sommer is the founder and president of Advance Publishing; Digital Cornerstone, a recording and video studio; and Reliable EDM, a precision machining company that specializes in electrical discharge machining. It is the largest company of its kind west of the Mississippi River (www.ReliableEDM.com). Two of his sons manage the EDM company, and another son manages his publishing company and recording studios which allows him to pursue his passion for writing.

Born in 1930, Sommer has been happily married since 1955 and has five children and 19 grandchildren. Sommer likes to read, and his hobbies are swimming and fishing. He exercises five times a week at home. Don't think of him as an old man. To this day Sommer regularly does 40 chin ups at one time. For his 78th birthday he tested himself and did 46 one-time chin ups. Twice a week he does dips at his kitchen corner countertop and chin-ups on a bar between his kitchen and garage. Three times a week he works out at a home gym and does push-ups and leg raises. Five times a week he walks on a treadmill for 20 minutes. He's in excellent health and has no plans to retire.

From Sommer's rich experiences and his passion to help students become successful, he is producing many new products that promote virtues and real-life skills.

1

The Challenge

This book is about sex, and I warn you, I'll be challenging you and speaking bluntly. I'll say things that are ugly and scary. So if you don't want to know the truth—DON'T READ THIS BOOK!

Youth are being constantly bombarded with stimulating sexual content on television, billboards, and the Internet, as well as in magazines, books, movies, video games, and music. Sexy teenage pop stars with their provocative clothing dance suggestively and sing lyrics that are sometimes violent. The promoters of these shows want kids to model these stars. The results? Millions of kids are imitating them without realizing the disastrous pitfalls that await them.

Multitudes of these sexually active young people are being infected each year with sexually transmitted diseases (STDs). Not only will these young people suffer from their initial infections, but many will suffer a lifetime of both physical and emotional difficulties. Will you become one of them?

If you're sexually active, there's an excellent chance you will get an STD. These diseases are not just humiliating and painful; they can also lead to infertility, cancer, and even death. In contrast, there are millions of youth who will never encounter these problems because they, and the person they will one day marry, made abstinence until marriage their choice. Unfortunately, many have abandoned their beliefs due to the false message of "safe" sex. What we need today is a new generation of youth who will challenge the teachings of "safe" sex and unashamedly declare their support for a lifestyle guaranteeing them a bright future.

This book is to help youth have a successful future. Some will listen; others will only listen after being hit on the head with a sledge hammer. My aim is to help youth avoid being clobbered. There needs to be an awareness of the many dangers of premarital sex and the tremendous benefits of abstinence until marriage. Let me say this loud and clear:

Abstinence Doesn't Mean Never Having Sex. It Means Saving Sex For Marriage.

You'll be reading stories and getting facts. But I warn you, some facts will be repulsive. "You're not scaring me!" you may say. "I'm living for maximum fun now!"

I'd answer, "Be foolish. Stuff cotton in your ears. Reject the truth and have your fun now. But remember, there's always tomorrow."

"Who cares about the future?"

"If you don't care about your future, then don't complain when your body is racked with pain and you suffer the rest of your life for your foolish decision to 'live for the now.'"

This Book Is for Intelligent Youth, Not for Dummies

This book is for intelligent youth, not for dummies. Some of you fell into the trap of today's foolish culture and engaged in premarital sex. You've been hoodwinked and burnt; you know it's wrong. You want to change. The good news is there's hope for you. Later we'll discuss this issue in "Renewed Purity."

Many teens have the "It can't happen to me" mentality concerning getting STDs. I've got bad news: It's happening, and at an alarming rate. Dr. Ray Bohlin, in "The Epidemic of Sexually Transmitted Diseases," stated: "Prior to 1960, there were only two significant sexually transmitted diseases: syphilis and gonorrhea. Both were easily treatable with antibiotics."[1]

But today The Associated Press reports that 1 in 4 teen girls has an STD, and "among those who admitted having sex, the rate was even more disturbing—40 percent had an STD."[2] What happened? Today our society is unconcerned about premarital sex; its primary concern is about the number of unwed pregnancies. Our society has falsely propagated that casual sex is okay as long as protections are used. This false message has caused STDs to flourish and brought untold tragedies to millions of teenagers and young adults. It's time to tell youth the truth.

I've written many award-winning children's books that teach children principles for successful living. Many children who read these books are today's youth. Their sex hormones are active, and if they make wrong decisions, their entire lives could be ruined.

I'm writing this book to counter the disastrous teachings about permissive sex in today's culture. I urge you to carefully consider your future. Remember, you won't remain a teenager forever. Don't think you can live any way you want without consequences. That's a fool's dream. Be intelligent. Think! The life you live now can lead to a bright or to a disastrous future. Don't endanger that future because of some dumb sexual decision you made in your youth. The aim of this book is to challenge and help you to live a happy and successful life.

Misconceptions, Myths, and Plain Lies About Sex

There are many misconceptions, myths, and plain lies about sex. The media distorts sex by portraying that as long as people are using protection and having fun, sex outside of marriage is normal and okay. Today premarital sex is also called recreational sex.

Many in our culture think youth are like animals, unable to control their passions. People ridicule abstinence until marriage as old-fashioned, unrealistic, unnatural, and unhealthy. They claim kids will be kids, and they'll have sex. So provide them with mountains of information on how to have "safe" sex. Follow these lies of our sex-saturated society, and you'll likely reap a lifetime of misery.

Today's Youth Aren't Animals

Today's young people aren't animals; they can control their passions. Over 50% of high school students claim they have never had sex. However, when these same high school students enter college, they face tremendous pressure to engage in casual sex. The media also increases this pressure by its unrealistic portrayal of sex and relationships. Today's youth are seldom shown the serious and fatal consequences of the sexual liberation movement. They've been hoodwinked.

Psychiatrist Fearful of Being Ostracized, Maligned, and Unemployed

Miriam Grossman, M.D., has been a psychiatrist at the University of California, Los Angeles (UCLA) Student Psychological Services for over 10 years, and has worked with students for over 20 years. She is the author of *Unprotected,*[3] a book that exposes the false and dangerous sexual advice students are provided in today's politically correct environment. She was so fearful the professional establishment would perceive her as being intolerant and then be ostracized and unemployed that she used "Dr. Anonymous" as her pen name. What a sad commentary on our so-called "tolerant" educational system when a trained psychiatrist must fear exposing the detrimental teachings taking place in today's schools.

Why did Grossman write such a book exposing the false teaching of "safe" sex? It's the same reason I'm writing this book. For years I've devoted my life to produce materials to train children for a life of success. Today, the advocates of "safe" sex promote a message that can lead youth to a lifetime of failure and suffering. The central teaching of "safe" sex is behaviors once considered destructive and immoral should now be taught as normal and natural. They teach casual sex is fine, even beneficial for mental health, so long as proper protection is used. However, Grossman reports, "On my campus, sexually active students are much more likely to seek counseling, and to rate their relationship as stressful."

Grossman tells about Olivia, an 18-year-old freshman who was the valedictorian of her senior class with hopes of going to medical school. When Olivia came to Grossman, she was vomiting up to six times a day. Olivia told about a short-lived relationship that resulted in her first experience with intimacy. "When it ended, it hurt so much," she said weeping. "I think about him all the time, and I haven't been going to one of my classes." Then she asked this piercing question, "Why do they tell you how to protect your body—from herpes and pregnancy—but they don't tell you what it does to your *heart*?"[4]

Grossman tells about Heather, a 19-year-old freshman. Heather came to Grossman because of her moodiness and crying spells. She finally told Grossman about a friend she really liked. Heather wanted to build a relationship with him, doing things like going shopping or seeing a movie together, but he just wanted to be with her and get his sexual benefits without bothering with a relationship. This so upset this normally upbeat and social freshman that she became withdrawn and filled with self-hate.[5]

In her book, *Unprotected*, Grossman writes:

> For those who trust academic journals more than Mom's wisdom, take a look at some recent research. In a study of 6,500 adolescents, sexually active teenage girls were more than three times more likely to be depressed, and nearly three times as likely to have had a suicide attempt, than girls who were not sexually active....
>
> Sure, there are women on campus who are making wise choices in their relationships. But if you think Heather and Olivia are unusual, I have news for you: our schedules are overbooked with them. They're lining

up for appointments and flooding our phone lines. I've seen so many students like these, they blur together in my mind, a pitiable crowd of confused, vulnerable young women, ill prepared for campus life, making poor choices, and paying high prices.

No amount of Prozac or Zoloft is going to solve this problem. These young women must, for their physical and emotional well-being, change their lifestyle.[6]

Are you listening? Can you picture this "pitiable crowd of confused, vulnerable young women, ill prepared for campus life, making poor choices, and paying high prices"? Remember, this is from a psychiatrist reporting from her years of personal experiences what's happening to many women who have listened to the detrimental teaching that there's no harm in casual sex as long as proper precautions are used.

Many men have no intention of having a serious relationship with their girlfriends. They use their girlfriends as free prostitutes. Many foolish women throw away their convictions and yield to the sexual advances of their boyfriends in hopes of satisfying their longing for love. Instead of finding a loving relationship they crave, many reap diseased bodies and broken hearts.

The sexually active often believe they only need to fear getting pregnant or getting an STD, but they're greatly mistaken. They don't realize the psychological and emotional problems that can accompany casual sex, or the haunting sense of being used and abused. It's time educators stop trying to be "politically correct" and tell students the truth about the detrimental effects of casual sex. What we need today are many more individuals like Grossman telling the truth regardless of the consequences from the politically correct.

Your Body Is Like an Expensive Car

Your body is like an expensive car. Would you put the cheapest oil into it or take care of it so it would give you years of excellent service? Life is a road trip. Are you looking for a life of cheap thrills and excitement that lead to failure, or will you plan for a successful future? Unfortunately, many youth feel empowered and throw off their shackles. In their so-called "freedom," they engage in behaviors that have serious consequences.

To be successful, you need short- and long-term goals for your life. Do you want to graduate? Do you want to have a career, be healthy, have a happy marriage, and raise a family? What must you do to achieve your goals? Plan your actions and write them down. Take a wrong turn, and you may have a head-on collision that will shatter all your goals.

If you had an expensive car, you'd take care of it. Why not do the same for your body? If you put junk into your body, what do you think will happen? It's obvious, you'll suffer for it. Youth tend to take risks. That's why auto insurance rates are so much higher for young drivers. Since sex is such a driving force in youth, many disregard the dangers and engage in risky behavior. Intelligent youth apply brakes to their turbocharged bodies in order to have a successful and happy future.

The First Rule for Success—Be Disciplined

The first rule for successful living is: Be disciplined! Look at successful athletes. How do they become successful? They practice discipline. Do you think that exercise and practice are always fun? They're not. Exercise and practice are hard work. But because great athletes are disciplined, they reap the fruits of their hard work.

Let's look at sex. Sex is beautiful, healthy, and good if experienced properly in marriage. We're programmed for sex. Between the ages of about 9 to 13, our bodies change. As a young kid, I had absolutely no use for girls; but one day things began to change. The opposite sex began looking attractive. That happens to all of us. It's natural.

Our sex hormones become extremely active in our teens, and we must be disciplined to avoid letting our passions destroy us. Sex is like fire. Controlled, it has tremendous benefits; uncontrolled, it's a disaster. With controlled fire we cook, heat our homes, drive our cars, and fly our jets. Uncontrolled, fire destroys our forests, homes, and lives.

Stand Up!

On June 25, 1950 the Korean War started. Sixteen months later I was ordered to report to Brooklyn for the draft. There the draft board had stamped on my papers, USMC (United States Marine Corp). I was sent to Parris Island, South Carolina, a plot of land 4 miles long and 3 miles wide. They took us new recruits and cut off our hair, gave every one of us a physical and new gear. They were going to make us into: "The Few. The Proud. The Marines!"

The first thing they taught us was discipline. In war you don't have time to debate. You must be trained to obey. Whatever the drill instructor (DI) said, we had to do. Period. We ate, slept, stood, marched, and ran whenever the DI gave the orders.

Parris Island is notorious for sand fleas. What do you do

when you're standing at attention and sand fleas land on your neck, face, and the back side of your hands sucking blood from you? You let them have their meal. Under no conditions will a DI let you swat them. The back of my hands and neck were swollen from the flea bites.

Picture a marine in the bushes crawling in the grass to attack an enemy. He must be quiet, otherwise he'll endanger the other marines with him. Marines must be brave and self-disciplined in order to become effective soldiers. When boot camp is over, the DI wants every marine to have discipline, pride, self-respect, and motivation to do his best. Every marine is trained to stand up straight and bear the motto of: "Semper Fidelis," Latin for "Always Faithful."

I'd like to enlist every one of you into the Marine Corp and put you through boot camp so you'd develop the guts to buck the crowd and stand up for what you know is right. Our country needs a new generation of wise, disciplined youth who will unashamedly expose and combat the destructive forces surrounding them both for themselves and for our nation.

Do you want a great future? Everyone does. The aim of this book is to ensure that you'll have a great future; it's not to make you miserable. Many young people see sex simply as an enjoyable physical act. But if the passion of sex is wrongly used, it can lead to emotional scars and devastating diseases that can destroy every plan you have for your future. I challenge you to stand up for what's right so you'll have a great future. Let's examine the battle youth face today.

2

The Battle

A boy sees a beautiful girl and is attracted to her. Hormones begin to work. "That's a beautiful girl," he says, "I'd like to meet her."

Inside the girl, something also stirs. She can't get the boy out of her mind. The girl says, "I hope he asks me out."

What's happening here? When we mature physically our sex hormones cause feelings of attraction and desire. It's perfectly normal. Now the battle begins, and this battle of controlling our hormones lasts a lifetime. How does one control sexual hormones?

Brandon Meets Ashley

Let's examine the life of two teenagers, Brandon and Ashley who both go to the same school. Ashley is an only child and at times gets lonely and longs for a relationship that will provide lasting friendship and acceptance. One day Ashley's and Brandon's eyes lock together, and there's a magnetic attraction. Brandon meets her in the cafeteria. In Ashley's heart, butterflies soar toward the heavens. She's in ecstasy. She can't get Brandon out of her mind. He's the answer to her dreams.

Brandon is also happy with Ashley, but he's young and has no desire to be strongly committed to a relationship. One thing Brandon does have—strong sexual urges. He knows that Ashley loves him, and he wants her to satisfy his ultimate desire—total sexual fulfillment.

They begin seeing each other. Ashley's parents work, so she's in the house alone after school. She invites Brandon over. They hug and kiss, but Brandon wants to do things that Ashley vowed never to do, She pushes him off.

Ashley Partially Yields

They continue to meet, but Brandon keeps pushing. If Ashley loses Brandon, her dream world will collapse. She can't let this happen. Ashley yields more of her body to Brandon, hoping to satisfy him and win his committed love. It repulses her, but she finally yields to Brandon and performs oral sex in order to make him happy.

Ashley feels guilty, but Brandon isn't satisfied. Ashley longs for a loving relationship; Brandon longs for a sexual relationship. Even though Ashley is becoming more and more depressed, she doesn't want to lose her lover. She still wants to remain a virgin, even though she has already violated parts of her vow of purity. She continues to push Brandon away. Finally, Brandon loses his patience and gives Ashley an ultimatum: "If you're not willing to make me happy and go all the way, I'll find someone else."

Ashley is in a dilemma. She wants to be a virgin, but she's deeply in love with Brandon. She can't stand the thought of losing him. Her problems before of loneliness and depression would seem like nothing if she lost Brandon. What should she do? The question gnaws at her insides.

Ashley Fully Yields

Brandon sees Ashley again. Terrified of losing him, Ashley finally breaks down and goes all the way. She hopes that yielding her body to Brandon will start a real love relationship. Brandon is delighted, but now when they see each other, he's only interested in sex. Ashley continues to long for a relationship. She continues to yield, but she's sinking deeper and deeper into a depression of guilt and shame. Her dream is turning into a nightmare.

One day Ashley discovers Brandon flirting with Nancy in school. She confronts him. "Why are you flirting with Nancy?"

Brandon brushes her off with, "So what?"

Ashley snaps back, "What do you mean, 'So what?'"

Brandon waves his hand and says, "You're jealous."

"Jealous," Ashley cries. "I thought you loved me."

"We'd better break off seeing each other," Brandon says as he casually walks away. "You're acting like you own me."

The Breakup

Ashley is crushed. Her world has shattered. She's been used and abused. She made a vow to be sexually abstinent until marriage, and now she's furious at herself. Over and over again she says, "How could I have been so stupid? My family and my church warned me to save sex for marriage, but I refused to listen.

"Why didn't I kick him out of the house when he began

pressuring me? I was warned over and over again how deceiving boys can be. I fell for his lies, and now I broke my vow. On top of that, he boasts to his friends that he had sex with me. Now my reputation is ruined."

What do we see happening between Brandon and Ashley? It's a battle faced by thousands. Everyone wants to be loved. Men aren't idiots. They know that women long for love, so they talk the language of love to get what they want.

Some think the way to find fulfillment in love is to do everything the other person desires. But true love is a respectful and shared experience. True love doesn't force one's will upon another. Brandon's concept of love was, "If you love me, you'll do what *I* want."

Are all guys like Brandon? Absolutely not. There are many decent young men. However, there are many guys just like Brandon. Brandon's love was selfish; he didn't care how Ashley felt. Ashley foolishly yielded in hopes of satisfying him. But Ashley discovered that even though she yielded, she never gained Brandon's true love.

3

The Dangers

Picture in your mind the most handsome boy or the most attractive girl. Imagine this boy or girl has a serious disease. When you examine their lips under a microscope you discover all sorts of ugly crawling creatures. Would you be interested in kissing these lips?

That's repulsive! Yes, it is. But I warned you not to read this book if you're not interested in truth. I'm not saying you'll get all kinds of diseases just from kissing, but I'm trying to make you realize that sex can expose you to all kinds of microscopic creatures that may cause you to get a sexually transmitted diseases (STDs).

Lifetime of Suffering

Some STDs can be cured, but some such as genital herpes, Human Papillomavirus (HPV), and Human Immunodeficiency Virus (HIV), which causes AIDS, have no cure. Some STDs that were once easily cured are now becoming resistant to some common antibiotics. Remember, sexual relations can be more than just intercourse whether vaginal or anal; it can also be oral-genital contact. From all of these one may get STDs. A person may look perfectly healthy on the outside, but still be infected.

One needs to realize that the sex organs of those engaging in casual sex may be filled with microscopic germs that can cause you a life-time of suffering. Do you understand what that means? As long as you live, you'll suffer. There's no cure!

Sex Is Fun

Is sex fun? Absolutely! Because it's so much fun, those engaging in it want more sex, and many are willing to take risks. However, engaging in premarital sex can be extremely dangerous. It's fun to drive a car fast—but getting an STD is like hitting a pole in a speeding car. You may survive, but you may also suffer a lifetime.

Just because you love someone doesn't mean that sex is okay. Sex may give you temporary pleasure, but it may result in pregnancy, disease, a broken heart, loss of respect, and ruined dreams. Those with self-respect refuse to give in to pressure. They know that true love does not equal sex; true love shows respect. If there's no respect, there's no true love.

Marriage is much more than having a sexual relationship. You have to be able to live with one another. There are many attractive women and handsome men, but not all of them make a suitable marriage partner. Some because of their vain and selfish attitudes would make a disastrous partner! In marriage, character is more important than appearance.

The same goes for dating. Here's an important bit of advice. When you date, be wise and seek someone with character and someone you can communicate with. Don't just focus on physical appearance.

Longing for Love

Deep within every man and woman is a longing to be loved. This dream person knocks on the door of your heart and you fantasize about your relationship. Your whole being pulsates with emotion. You're in love. Your hopes are high to build a lasting romance. You talk and laugh together in hopes of learning more about your lover, for that's the objective of romance. Romance deals with communication; it's something every woman desires.

But along this road of finding this someone to fulfill this longing of love are many dangerous traps. Unfortunately, many become ensnared and never find love's ultimate fulfillment.

Deception and Heartache

Let's look at a girl who was raised by a single mother. We'll call her Amber. Amber's mother got pregnant twice as a teenager. Now she's busy with her full-time job at a food market checkout counter and with trying to meet the needs of her two children. Amber's mother tries to do her best, but Amber is always home alone after school taking care of her younger brother.

Amber knows about the dangers of sex from her "safe" sex instruction classes. Amber is well-developed and attractive, and many boys are interested in her. She loves the attention. One day she meets Troy, an older teen. He's athletic and handsome, and all Amber's friends are attracted to him. Out of all the girls, Troy asks Amber for a date. Amber feels honored and is thrilled.

In Amber's circle of friends, they talk freely about sex. Amber has no intentions of being a virgin. She plans to practice "safe" sex.

Amber has high expectations for herself. She gets good

grades and wants to go to college and become a nurse. Then she plans on getting married and having a family. One sure thing, she doesn't want to end up like her mother. However, Amber wants to have lots of fun. She believes in the message of "safe" sex: limit your partners and always use a condom.

There's no question that limiting partners decreases the risk of STDs. But what Amber doesn't realize is if she limits her partners to just two, and each of the two had ten previous partners, she has in effect had sexual contact with twenty people!

As the star school athlete, Troy had numerous sexual relationships with girls. Troy and Amber began dating and having sexual relations. Unknown to Troy, he has an HPV virus.

HPV (human papillomavirus) is a virus that is spread through skin-to-skin contact, sexual contact, anal sex, and oral sex. There are over 100 different HPV viruses. At least 30 types of HPV cause different types of cancer. In an article on "How common is HPV?" the Centers for Disease Control and Prevention states:

> Approximately 20 million people are currently infected with HPV, and another 6.2 million Americans become newly infected each year. At least 50 percent of sexually active men and women acquire genital HPV infection at some point in their lives.[1]

Odds are if you're sexually active, you'll get this disease.

Currently, there is no cure for HPV. Amber contracted HPV from Troy. Unknown to Amber, a condom doesn't guarantee full protection against HPV. Condoms don't cover the skin surrounding the genitals and anus where the virus is active. Even if there is no penetration, if there's skin-to-skin contact, there's a risk of getting this disease.

Genital warts are usually soft and flesh colored. They appear around the sexual area of males and females. In females, warts may appear even inside the vagina. Though genital warts can be successfully treated, they may reappear at any time, calling for another round of treatment. There are also types of HPV that cause cervical cancer in women, and if left untreated may lead to an early death.

Since there's no cure for HPV, Amber may have this infection for a long time and spread it to others. Imagine the stigma when it gets around she has this disease. You can rest assured she won't be the school's most popular girl.

Sexual Past Comes Back to Haunt

Stephen Reynolds writing in *Reader's Digest* says, "I was in my 40s, with a young son, and my wife and I were building a life around him. That's when something from my past threatened to take it all away."

The past threatening his future was from his previous sexual encounters. Reynolds had a graduate degree and was a business strategist in the technology industry. He had never smoked, yet he was diagnosed with lung cancer.

Reynolds reports: "Maura Gillison, MD, a researcher and

professor at Johns Hopkins University in Baltimore, was among the first to study the link between the growth of head and neck cancers among younger nonsmokers and certain types of the sexually transmitted human papillomavirus (HPV). It's the same virus that causes the majority of cervical cancers and warts. The risks are scary because the virus is really common, even in teenagers...Of the more that 35,000 people who will be diagnosed with oral cancer this year, 25 percent of us will connect our diagnosis to HPV infection."

Reynolds describes his painful experiences dealing with the operation to remove the cancer and his chemo treatments. They provide a feeding tube to help him in eating. "They tell me that I can put a Big Mac in a blender," he says, "grind it up with protein shakes, and pour it all into the tube."

He struggles not to use the feeding tube, and his treatments leave him so frail. He longs to play with his son, but there are times, "I just don't have it and fall asleep in the middle of giving him a horsey ride," he says. "My poor wife. My poor kid. All I have the energy to do is lie still and try not to bother them."

In a side note on HPV and You, *Readers Digest* brings out this fact: "One type of HPV raises the risk of oral cancer by 3,200 percent."[2]

Beware of Alcohol and Drugs

Alcohol and drugs pose another danger that can lead young people into unwanted premarital sex. *Daily Mail,* in "The true cost of sex under 16," tells what happened to a young woman:

The night Clare Gibbons lost her virginity was unforgettable. Not because it was special or romantic or even exciting-but precisely because it was anything but.

At the tender age of 14, she and a friend went to an older boy's house for the evening. Both girls agreed to camp in the garden overnight with the 19-year-old and his friend.

"We all thought it would be fun," she recalls. Then the drinking began and before she knew it, Clare was lying beneath the canvas having sex with a man she barely knew. It was a sickening experience which will be etched on her memory for ever.

"I can remember what happened," says Clare, now a 17-year-old media studies student. "But I was in such a tipsy daze I was powerless to stop it. The next morning, I could barely look at him. I felt absolutely sick, and so used and dirty."[3]

Clare's experience "was a sickening experience that will be etched on her memory forever." Sex produces some of life's most powerful emotions.

Blount Nurses for Health Education tells about another girl who went to the lake with her boyfriend. Curious, she tried a can of beer. She drank some more until she passed out. Her boyfriend raped her. Embarrassed, she didn't tell anyone. Her plan to remain a virgin until marriage was shattered. Her ex-boyfriend boasted to all his friends that he had sex with her. Now instead of being respected, she became known as "easy."[4]

Healthy People 2010 in the article on "Sexually Transmitted Diseases" stated: "Many studies document the association of substance abuse, especially the abuse of alcohol and drugs, with STDs."[5]

Internet, Chat Rooms, Instant Messaging

Many youth are unaware of the dangers of putting personal information on the Web. They put their names, addresses, phone numbers, school, and pictures of themselves on the Web without proper safeguards. They believe they're just sharing information with their friends, but the world is also watching.

Many are lonely and looking for friends, but they don't realize they are attracting sharks—sexual predators acting as friends. These predators are masters of saying what you long to hear, but they're after one thing—to exploit your loneliness so they can abuse you sexually. They begin to chat, and many youth fantasize and share personal information and even pictures of themselves. These sharks appear kind and tender and may even offer gifts. Some engage in sexual discussions in the chat rooms, instant messages, and emails.

What many youth don't realize is the person they are chatting with may be a disguised predator looking to fulfill his sexual drives—voluntarily or forcibly. There are also homosexual predators. These predators might send pictures of a handsome young boy or gorgeous girl, but it's all a farce. When the victims meet this dream young person, they're shocked to find an older person. Now they're trapped and helpless before a powerful individual. To avoid identification, and knowing that dead people don't talk, some sexual predators kill their victims after raping them.

Beware! Don't be gullible and become a victim! Inform your parents. If you must correspond, use a non-gender screen name. Never provide any personal information online: real name, personal picture, home telephone or cell phone numbers, school, address, passwords, social security number, etc. Never accept any downloads from strangers or meet anyone you don't know. Keep in mind: today's chatrooms are the hunting grounds for sexual predators. Protect yourself—don't become a victim!

Beware! Never Share Personal Information Online. Remember, The World Is Able To Watch.

4

Sexually Transmitted Diseases

What makes sex so dangerous? One of the reasons sex is so dangerous is youth trained in "safe" sex often feel like supermen or superwomen resulting in an epidemic of sexually transmitted diseases where millions of new infections are occurring every year. Many youth today have no fear from sex.

I've got bad news for you. One microscopic STD bug can enter your system and cause a lifetime of suffering and pain. Getting one of these bugs can cause genital warts or cancer. Another bug can cause genital painful sores and ulcers. Yet another bug can lead to female infertility, forever destroying any dream of bringing children into the world.

If you refuse to abstain from sex until marriage—a foolish course—condoms do offer some physical protection. But they offer no protection from guilt, heartaches, disappointments, and shame. Some falsely promote condoms as the magic cure, but condoms aren't totally safe. Some fail; and some STDs, such as herpes, HPV, and syphilis, are spread by skin-to-skin contact, so these diseases aren't stopped by condoms. Remember, condoms offer "risk reduction," not "risk elimination."

Let's look at two teenagers, Jennifer and Brian. Think of Jennifer's emotions when she yielded her virginity to Brian and a month later developed painful blisters around her sexual area. When she went to the doctor she learned she had herpes, an incurable disease affecting millions!

Brian had two previous sexual encounters which infected

him with herpes. Brian happened to be asymptomatic, meaning he had no symptoms but still carried the infection. Jennifer, however, had flu-like symptoms and repeated painful blisters. Three months later, Brian and Jennifer broke up.

The virus in Jennifer traveled to the sensory nerves of the spinal cord. Even when the symptoms disappeared, the virus remained inside her nerve cells. Now new sores and blisters may appear periodically and cause painful urination.

When Jennifer finds another boyfriend, she faces another problem. Should she immediately tell her new boyfriend about her incurable disease, should she wait until they are serious, or should she never say anything? Jennifer knows that one day she has to reveal what happened to her. Imagine the emotional impact when Jennifer breaks the news to the person she hopes to marry.

If Jennifer had another chance, do you think she'd make a firm commitment to remain sexually pure until marriage?

Oral Sex

Picture this scenario. You vow to abstain from sex until marriage. You go to a party and some boys and girls begin fooling around. Some of them engage in oral sex. One of the girls tells you, "Oral sex isn't sex. It's just having fun."

"Okay," you tell yourself, "I can do that and still be a virgin."

A few days later your throat is sore. "It's strep throat," you tell yourself.

But your sore throat doesn't go away. You visit the doctor

and he says, "You have gonorrhea of the throat."

You're shocked and devastated. You thought that oral sex was risk-free, but you discover you were dead wrong. Marla Kushner, a physician who runs a school-based adolescent health clinic in Chicago, says, "Kids come in thinking they have strep." Then when they discover they have gonorrhea of the throat, "they're grossed out—and they're devastated. They have no idea that these sorts of things even exist."[1]

Kids would be grossed out if their friend took the bubble gum out of their mouth and offered it to them. A typical reaction would be, "Are you crazy! You want me to put in my mouth something you chewed on?" Yet many do something much worse—they do oral sex!

There's a great misconception about oral sex. It is not safe. You can't get pregnant, but you're a candidate for a wide variety of STDs. Some of these STDs from oral sex are incurable! Bernadine Healy, M.D., in *U.S. News & World Report* on "Clueless About Risks of Oral Sex" states:

> To some young people, oral sex preserves virginity—technically speaking—and allows for what is perceived as risk-free sexual intimacy. From a medical perspective, however, this *is* sex—and, generally, unsafe sex. People seem clueless that sexually transmitted diseases such as herpes, gonorrhea, chlamydia, and human papillomavirus can take hold in parts of the oral cavity during sex with infected partners and that STD-ridden mouths are likely to transmit disease to uninfected genitals. HPV

is a particularly scurrilous threat, since it incubates silently in the back of the mouth and is now linked to a dangerous form of throat cancer in both men and women similar to the one that arises in the cervix.[2]

Imagine if you discovered you had an STD. What should you do? The right thing to do is to contact all your previous partners and tell them the news. Not very exciting, is it? It certainly wouldn't be great for your popularity! If you happen to get a viral STD, then you're really in big trouble since many are incurable. It could be with you the rest of your life causing you misery and pain.

Message of ABC

School health providers expose the risks of overeating and poor nutrition, a sedentary lifestyle, lack of exercise, smoking, drugs, binge and chronic drinking, sun exposure, and wearing seat belts. But when it comes to sex, they promote the risky behavior of ABC, another name for "safe" sex, instead of promoting the only sure method for avoiding all STDs: abstinence from all sexual activity, including vaginal, oral, and anal sex.

The popular ABC message is:

A—Abstinence: Practice abstinence by delaying sex.

B—Be Faithful: If you can't restrain yourself, be faithful to one partner or reduce your partners.

C—Use Condoms: Practice correct and consistent condom use.

Here's the instruction of one "safe" sex advocate: "To help prevent both pregnancy and STIs [sexual transmitted infections], you should correctly and consistently use a birth control method like the Pill, contraceptive injection or diaphragm (for pregnancy prevention) and a condom (to prevent STIs)."[3]

Many health providers mention abstinence as being 100% effective for the prevention of STDs and pregnancies, but then go into great detail about on how to have "safe" sex. In a nonjudgmental atmosphere they describe the many sexual methods. They stress if you happen to get pregnant, the earlier you have an abortion the better.

What message do many students take home when they receive the ABC instruction? Yes, abstinence is a safe method for STD prevention, but casual sex is also safe as long as proper precautions are used. The results? I'll let the Centers for Disease Control and Prevention (CDC) from the Department of Health and Human Services state what's happening:

Sexually transmitted diseases (STDs) remain a major public health challenge in the United States. While substantial progress has been made in preventing, diagnosing, and treating certain STDs in recent years, CDC estimates that 19 million new infections occur each year, almost half of them among young people ages 15 to 24. In addition to the physical and psychological consequences of STDs, these diseases also exact a tremendous economic toll. Direct medical costs associated with STDs in the United States are estimated at up to $14.1 billion annually.[4]

The Associated Press reports, "In the first study of its kind, researchers at the federal Centers for Disease Control and Prevention found at least one in four teenage American girls has a sexually transmitted disease. The most common one is a virus that can cause cervical cancer, and the second most common can cause infertility. Nearly half the black teens in the study had at least one sexually transmitted infection....Among those who admitted having sex, the rate was even more disturbing — 40 percent had an STD."[5]

Do these figures concern you? Or must you become one of the STD statistics before you listen and groan over your foolish decision? There are over 25 STDs, including bacterial vaginosis, chlamydia, genital herpes, gonorrhea, hepatitis B, HIV/AIDS, genital warts, syphilis, and trichomoniasis. I'm not going to describe all these diseases, for this book is about prevention. But let's look at some of the symptoms.

Some STDs may cause pain or burning when urinating; itching; swollen glands in the genital area; pain in the legs, buttocks, back, or abdomen; loss of appetite; weight loss; nausea; vomiting; diarrhea; headaches; sore throat; muscle aches; fever; extreme fatigue; blisters; skin turning yellow, red, brown, or purplish inside mouth, nose, or eyelids; skin rash; warts in the genital area; bleeding between menstrual periods; and open sores on the penis or vagina. Besides the serious health effects of STDs, there's also the cost for treating these infections, and some need lifetime treatment. Contracting an STD can alter your life forever.

C. Everett Koop, M.D., former U.S. Surgeon General, revealed this startling fact, "When you have sex with someone, you are having sex with everyone they have had sex with for the last ten years, and everyone they and their partners have had sex with for the last ten years."

In other words, your sex partner may be carrying the germs from any other sex partners down the line. That's how infections spread and grow. If you engage in casual sex, the silent transmission of disease-causing viruses or bacteria may make you a victim.

Superbugs

Over sixty years ago, Dr. Alexander Fleming discovered the first widely used antibiotic, penicillin. For decades, doctors have been prescribing antibiotics to combat various diseases. But now scientists are warning us that the overuse of antibiotics has created another serious problem—superbugs.

Here's what happens. At first the antibiotic kills practically all the germs. However, a few survive. These few are weakened, but they survive the attack from the antibiotic. These weakened germs reproduce. Again the antibiotic is used and kills most of them, but again some survive. The survivors are more resistant to the antibiotic than before. This process continues until we have "superbugs," bacteria that are totally resistant to antibiotics.

One of the sexually transmitted diseases that has joined the ranks of superbugs is gonorrhea. This disease can leave men and women infertile and places them at a higher risk of getting AIDS. *USA Today* in the article "Gonorrhea mutates to resist antibiotic treatment" reports: "Gonorrhea has become so resistant to one class of antibiotics that the Centers for Disease

Control and Prevention announced Thursday that the drugs should no longer be used to treat it."[6]

AIDS

Let's examine one STD that is constantly in the news, the global epidemic HIV/AIDS (Human Immunodeficiency Virus/Acquired Immune Deficiency Syndrome). Avert, an international AIDS charity, reports, "More than 25 million have died of AIDS since 1981." They say that today, approximately 33 million people are living with HIV/AIDS, and "young people (under 25 years old) account for half of all new HIV infections worldwide."[7]

If you're not interested in statistics, consider how you'd feel if a family member were one of those 25 million who had died of AIDS; or if you were slowly dying of the virus.

People don't "catch" AIDS. They become infected with HIV, which leads to AIDS. Most people get HIV from having sex with someone infected or from taking drugs where a needle contaminated with the virus was used. You may have the virus and not even know it, or you may get some symptoms that you dismiss as the flu. Once infected with the virus, though, you become a carrier who can pass unknowingly HIV to others. Remember, you can get the virus after only one sexual encounter with an infected person.

For ten years you may think you're healthy, but the virus slowly wears down your immune system so it loses its ability to fight infection. If you are like most people, then your immune system becomes so severely weakened that HIV becomes AIDS. One type of white blood cell, called a CD4 cell, drops from a normal level of about 500 to 1,200 per microliter of blood to less than 200 cells per microliter of blood. Now your body loses its ability to fight infections and certain cancers. You become sick. You go to the doctor and he tells you the shocking news, "You have AIDS!"

Some AIDS patients die quickly. Others survive for years by taking powerful medication for the rest of their lives, sometimes with unpleasant side effects. In spite of the world's best medical efforts, **THERE'S NO CURE FOR AIDS!**

The U.S. government's Centers for Disease Control and Prevention states: "In the United States, HIV infection and AIDS have had a tremendous effect on men who have sex with men (MSM)." In one year, "MSM accounted for 71% of all HIV infections among male adults and adolescents….In a recent CDC study of young MSM, 77% of those who tested HIV-positive mistakenly believed that they were not infected." And "MSM as a group continues to be the population most affected by HIV infection and AIDS."[8]

One wonders how anyone can advocate such a destructive behavior when "MSM [homosexuals] accounted for 71% of all HIV infections among male adults and adolescents." In addition to the problems of HIV infection and AIDS, the Centers for Disease Control and Prevention says: "Gay male adolescents are two to three times more likely than their peers to attempt suicide."[9] Oxford University's "International Journal of Epidemiology" said in their concluding remarks: "Life expectancy at age 20 years for gay and bisexual men is 8 to 20 years less than for all men. If the same pattern of mortality were to continue, we estimate that nearly half of gay and bisexual men currently aged 20 years will not reach their 65th birthday."[10]

In western societies where AIDS patients receive better care and drugs, there emerges another problem. Mark Wainberg, an AIDS researcher, activist, and former president of the International AIDS Society, directs the McGill University AIDS Center at the Montreal Jewish Hospital. In the article, "A dark side to good news of living longer with HIV," Wainberg says, "People who have been HIV-positive over long periods are presenting in high numbers with a variety of cancers that are both life-threatening and that defy the traditional therapies used to treat cancer in those who do not have HIV."[11]

Am I trying to scare you? You'd be a fool not to be scared. Think! Are a few moments of pleasure worth suffering from an incurable disease the rest of your life? And if that's not enough to scare you, some STDs can make both men and women infertile. You'd *never* be able to bring a child into the world!

Remember: All it takes is one sexual act with an infected person to get a sexually transmitted disease.

Fear of Getting STDs

Is it rational for an individual to choose a path of abstinence because he or she is afraid of getting an STD? Is a boy or girl who practices abstinence from all sexual activity stupid because he or she realizes that there are over 25 STDs they can be infected with? And if they get HIV, it may be irreversible and last a lifetime. If a girl gets Human Papillomavirus (HPV), she may develop cancer; if she gets chlamydia, she may become infertile. Her dreams for a happy future can be shattered with just one sexual encounter. If anyone cares about their future, it's a very intelligent decision to be fearful of getting an STD.

"Safe" Sex Message in a Nutshell

Here's the "safe" sex message in a nutshell. Sex is natural, but when you have sex, use protection. If you get an STD, see a doctor right away. If you get pregnant, the sooner you get an abortion the safer it is.

A strong message of "safe" sex is to always use a condom when engaging in sex. Planned Parenthood, one of the leading advocates for "safe" sex, provides contraceptives and abortions for women who have undesired pregnancies. You'd think that since they're so concerned about girls becoming pregnant they would provide them with the best protection.

Consumer Reports, a non-profit organization that scientifically tests and rates thousands of products, tested 23 condoms. Two of the worst condoms tested were from Planned Parenthood! In addition, the only two condoms to receive a "Poor" rating came from Planned Parenthood.[12] It's rather strange that Planned Parenthood, an advocate of "safe sex," and claim on their website to be "America's most trusted provider of reproductive health care," provides the lowest quality condoms. The question arises: Is Planned Parenthood really interested in protecting kids?

This is what psychiatrist Miriam Grossman, who counseled over 2,000 university students, writes in her book *Unprotected*:

Tell them [young people] we're waging a war against these bugs, and the bugs are winning. Tell them 20 million people in our country have HPV, mostly women and minorities, and that doctors, drug companies, and corporations are making billions. Tell them this contributes to skyrocketing health insurance. Tell them their behavior, and their friends, can make a difference. Tell them the truth!

A delusion is "a false belief that is resistant to reason or confrontation with actual fact." I submit that "safer sex" is a delusion, one that especially imperils young women on campus. We need to come clean, and fully disclose to our youth the dreadful consequences of behaviors encouraged by our culture, so they can make fully informed decisions. The only people who are completely safe are those who, along with their spouses, waited for marriage, and once married, remain faithful. The ones who are "safer" delay sexual behavior, discriminate carefully in their choice, and understand the weight of their decisions.[13]

Are you listening to what psychiatrist Grossman says?

"'Safer sex' is a delusion."

What is the true safe sex message according to Grossman? "The only people who are completely safe are those who, along with their spouses, waited for marriage, and once married, remain faithful."

Controlling Sexual Desires

It's universally taught that unless the woman consents to sex, the male has to control his sexual passion. If he refuses, he's imprisoned on rape charges. Likewise sexual predators of children are a plague in our society. These beasts refuse to repress their passions and insist on fulfilling their sexual urges with whoever they want. Sexual predators are universally condemned and imprisoned.

When a female dog is in heat, you can be certain any male dogs in the vicinity will try to mount her. We don't fault the dogs when they see a dog in heat and want to mount her. But youth aren't animals who must follow every instinct. We should have higher expectations for today's youth. They're human beings who can control their behavior.

Millions of youth today understand the dangers of STDs and refuse to believe the lie that "Everyone's having sex." They are controlling their sexual desires and saying loud and clear, "NO!" to all premarital sex. Those making this decision will reap a lifetime of rewards.

Some Claim Sexual Repression Is Unnatural, Abnormal, and Repressive

Some "safe" sex advocates claim that striving to be a virgin and refusing to engage in sex before marriage is unnatural, abnormal, and repressive. However, those same "safe" sex advocates say condoms should always be used when having sex. But isn't using a condom also unnatural, abnormal, and repressive?

When a man has a sexual urge, shouldn't he have the right to do what's natural and not repress his desire? If he sees a woman or a child, should he repress his sexual desire? It's obvious he must. No man has a license to satisfy his sexual desire every time he's aroused. If he does, it's called rape. There's universal outrage against anyone who does not control his sexual impulses.

Passions are a powerful force within us. Passion isn't love; it's a fleeting feeling of emotional excitement. If uncontrolled, it can destroy us. By venting their passions, many have made the disastrous decisions to rape their victims.

Rape is not always caused by strangers. About half of the persons raped knew their attackers. To loosen inhibitions, rapists often use alcohol and mix drugs into drinks so their victim blacks out and can't remember what happened. If you happen to be a victim, report the incident immediately to the police and preserve all evidence. Go straight to an emergency room. They have medical personnel trained to take care of rape victims.

The world's jails are full of men who tried forcing their sexual urges on men, women, and children. To say restraining sexual impulses is unnatural, abnormal, and repressive is absurd. Societies worldwide put restrictions on sexual expressions.

"What am I going to do?" you ask. "I'm burning inside to vent my sexual passions."

There are two options—either you act on or control your sexual impulses. Remember:

Sex Without Consent Is Rape!

5

Pregnancy and Abortion

L et's imagine a teenage girl named Emily who is deeply in love with Bob. She's been dating Bob for a while, and one day in a highly charged moment she breaks down and yields to Bob's sexual advances. The barrier is broken. Both have been taught about "safe" sex and try to use all the safe procedures they learned. They believe they can continue to safely experiment for a more satisfying sexual experience. They don't realize, though, that some of the "safe" sex practices fail.

You're Pregnant!

One day Emily notices she missed her regular period. She goes to the doctor and he announces, "You're pregnant!"

Emily's world falls apart. She's overwhelmed with despair, guilt, shame, and confusion. "I can't believe this happened to me!" she groans over and over again. "What did we do wrong?"

Questions and thoughts race through her mind, "What shall I do? I'm too young to have a baby. What will my parents, relatives, and friends say? Should I have an abortion? Is it right to have an abortion and destroy an unborn child? How am I going to pay for all the needs of a baby? Should I give up the baby for adoption? Why did this happen to me?"

Counselor's Advice

Emily visits a counselor. "You're too young and immature for a child," the counselor advises. "Two out of three teenage mothers live in poverty. Many teenage mothers drop out of school and have limited social opportunities. Your life as a mother will be dramatically different. No longer will you be able to do the things you want. Your child will determine your limits.

"Besides, babies are expensive. As a parent you'll spend much of your time taking care of the baby and making ends meet. You'll have a living baby with you that needs to be fed, changed, and constantly taken care of. You'll need to provide food, clothing, diapers, baby furniture, and health care. Taking care of a baby requires 24 hours a day, 7 days a week. Your life will never be the same.

"I encourage you to have an abortion. The fetus is just a blob of tissue. If you do it now, no one will ever know you're pregnant. Abortions aren't dangerous; they'll use gentle suction to end your pregnancy."

Emily leaves the counselor confused and depressed. "I don't want to destroy this baby," she tells herself. "What should I do?"

Get Married

Emily likes Bob, but she doesn't love Bob enough to want to marry him. She was just having fun dating. But now that she's pregnant, she thinks, "Maybe Bob and I can get married and raise the child together."

Emily breaks the news to Bob and says, "I'm pregnant."

"What!"

"I'm pregnant."

"Are you sure you're going to have a baby?"

"I've been tested by the doctor."

Bob doesn't want a baby. He's a teenager and plans to go to college. Having a baby would ruin his career plans. Bob has a simple solution, "Emily, you MUST get an abortion!"

"I can't kill my baby!" Emily says as tears begin to flow.

"It's not a baby, it's a fetus!" Bob says, trying to convince her to have an abortion. "The fetus becomes a human only after it's born."

"That's not true. You even called it a 'baby.' It's a growing human being that shouldn't be killed. If I killed my unborn child, I'd be committing murder."

"That's pure nonsense! You MUST get an abortion."

"Why don't we get married?"

"Are you crazy? I'm too young to get married. I'm going to college."

"Please! Let's give it a try. I'll make going to college easy for you. I'll get a job and support you while you go to school."

"Sorry," Bob says as he leaves. "There's no way I'm getting married. You have a very simple solution. Get an abortion. If you don't, you'll have to take care of the baby by yourself. Don't count on me!"

The door slams, and Emily is alone. Bob promised over and over again how he loved her and wanted her to be part of his life forever. In the heat of passion she believed him. But now that she's pregnant, he's gone.

Bob tells his close friend, Troy, "I got Emily pregnant, and she refuses to get an abortion."

"Do you realize that you'll be paying child support until the child is 18 years old," Troy reminds him, "and maybe through college, too?"

"Wow! I never thought of that."

"I work with a guy that got a girl pregnant in another state, and every week the company takes money out of his paycheck to pay for the child. Whatever you do, you'd better get her to abort that baby."

"Thanks for the advice."

Bob asks himself, "What can I do to get Emily to abort the baby?" Suddenly he gets an idea. "I know what I'll do!"

The next day he calls Emily on the phone and says in a loving voice, "Emily, I'm sorry for being harsh with you the other day. Please forgive me."

"I forgive you." A ray of hope fills Emily's depressed spirit.

"I've been doing a lot of thinking. You want to get married?"

"Yes! By all means!" Emily's heart glimmers with hope. "Then we can have the baby together."

"Listen carefully to what I have to say," Bob says in a sweet loving voice. "I sincerely love you, Emily, and I really want to marry you. But I don't want us to start married life with a baby. Why don't we abort this baby? When I graduate from high school, we'll get married. Then after awhile when we can afford it, we'll have another baby."

"Bob, I can't abort this baby," Emily says with tears flowing down her cheeks. "I've been raised in church, and I know deep within me it's wrong to kill an unborn baby."

Bob is worried. Emily isn't responding to his plan. "Listen Emily, you won't have to pay anything for the abortion. I'll pay for it. And no one will know about it, not even your parents."

"I have to live with my conscience, Bob. I'll be murdering my child. I can't live like that. I already violated what I was taught in my church by having sex with you. I can't make matters worse. Please, let's get married."

The Ultimatum

"Ohhhh!" groans Bob to himself. "She's also one of those religious freaks." Then Bob says very firmly, "Emily, you have my word. I'll marry you *only* if you get an abortion. Do you understand? I *refuse* to marry you if you defy me by having the baby. That's final!" Bob slams the phone down.

Emily is crushed. She knows Bob can't be trusted; he's lied to her in the past. She now suffers daily with bouts of guilt, shame, depression, and despair. Emily curses the day she yielded to Bob's sexual advances. Now she's alone, pregnant, and has to make decisions on what to do. After many agonizing weeks, Emily finally comes to the conclusion, "I'd rather suffer the shame of being pregnant, than suffer the guilt of murdering my baby. When the baby comes, I'll either keep it or let it be adopted so it can have a good home."

Listen to the plea of another girl who became pregnant.

I'm a high school senior. I got pregnant before I was 14 and had my baby at 14. I never considered abortion because of my religious beliefs. I love my little boy and

I'm so proud of him. But, I can't tell you how hard it has been to attend classes, try to study some, and care for him. I can't even think about going to college. My sister is a junior in my high school. I'm really happy she hasn't gotten pregnant, but sometimes I'm jealous of her. She goes out on dates, attends games and proms, and does all of the fun things I should have been able to do, while I stay home taking care of my little boy. I lost my youth because of a few minutes I spent with a guy in the back seat of his car. He won't even speak to me now! How I wish I could have those few minutes back so that I could have my youth back! Don't make the same mistake I made! PLEASE![1]

Teen Pregnancy

Some girls see Hollywood stars becoming pregnant and become seduced into thinking it's no big deal. They think if celebrities can become pregnant and proudly display their baby bumps, so can they. *Time* magazine in "Children Having Children," reports the reality:

As infants, the offspring of teen mothers have high rates of illness and mortality. Later in life, they often experience educational and emotional problems. Many are victims of child abuse at the hands of parents too immature to understand why their baby is crying or how their doll-like plaything has suddenly developed a will of its own. Finally, these children of children are prone to dropping out and becoming teenage parents themselves....

Pregnancy is widely viewed as the very hub of the U.S. poverty cycle. "A lot of the so-called feminization of poverty starts off with teenagers' having babies," says Lucile Dismukes of the Council on Maternal and Infant Health in Atlanta, a state advisory group. "So many can't rise above it to go back to school or get job skills."[2]

In the same article, *Time* presents this scene:

It is early afternoon, and the smells of dirty diapers and grease mingle in the bleak Minneapolis apartment. The TV is tuned to All My Children, and Stephanie Charette, 17, has collapsed on the sofa. Her rest is brief. Above the babble of the actors' voices comes a piercing wail. Larissa, her three-week-old daughter, is hungry. In an adjacent bedroom, Joey, 1 ½ years old and recovering from the flu, starts to stir...

It was an "accident," she explains. So too was her second baby. "I'm always tired," she laments, "and I can't eat." Before Joey's birth, before she dropped out of school, Stephanie dreamed of being a stewardess. Now her aspirations are more down-to-earth. "I want to pay my bills, buy groceries and have a house and furniture. I want to feel good about myself so my kids can be proud of me." It has been a long, long while, she confides, "since I had a good time."[3]

Wake up teenagers! Getting pregnant will dramatically alter your future in ways you haven't planned. Many propose the solution to prevent teen pregnancy is abortion. But that's not the solution. The solution is abstain from sex until you're married. It's 100 percent effective in preventing pregnancies.

Post-Abortion Stress

Miriam Grossman, M.D., in her book *Unprotected* tells about 19-year-old Kelly who knew a boy just for one week. They went to a party, drank too much, and engaged in sex using protection. Kelly had no fear when her period was late, for the boy had used a condom. She went to get examined and the nurse told her she was pregnant. Something must have happened to the condom.

Kelly went to Planned Parenthood. The counselor assured her both surgical and medical abortions were many times safer than giving birth and psychological problems were rare. Kelly had the abortion and felt relieved it was over. But now she feels sad, guilty, and alone.[4] Grossman asks:

> Now I don't know if Kelly will end up with long-term symptoms or not, but why is there an *assumption* she'll be fine? Why does student health not schedule a postabortion follow-up, to check on how she is coping? Why are women like Kelly sent home from Planned Parenthood knowing what to do in case of fever or heavy bleeding, but without a number to call or a Web site to visit if she is distressed? And why, if she is seen in the future at the campus counseling center, will she surely

be asked whether she was ever beaten or neglected by her parents, but not if she ever had an abortion?[5]

Grossman goes on to tell about the website www.afterabortion.com where women can seek help after an abortion. The website states: "We don't allow discussion of prolife or prochoice views or issues here."[6] It's open only to women who had an abortion so they can chat with other women and try to find answers and comfort from their disturbing abortion experiences. Grossman goes into details about the sufferings some of these women encounter because of their abortions. Then she reports:

As a psychiatrist, what do I learn from this Web site? First, I see in these women what I see in many of my patients—exceptional strength and courage. They continue to function, even with their hideous flashbacks and raw emotions....Second, many women here have textbook cases of PTSD [Post-Traumatic Stress Disorder]. Some have severe cases, and would benefit from therapy and medication. A few are hopeless and suicidal, and sound to me to be in need of hospitalization.

It's disturbing that these women are neglected by mainstream mental health. I am dismayed to learn they have nowhere to turn but a Web site. I am alarmed that girls and women being prepared for abortion are left unaware of the possible scenarios ahead of them.[7]

This is what *Ms. Magazine* had to say on their website about post-abortion stress disorder:

Sounds scientific, but don't be fooled—it's a made-up term. Not recognized as an official syndrome or diagnosis by the American Psychiatric Association, the American Psychological Association, or any other mainstream authority, it is a bogus affliction invented by the religious right. Those who claim its existence define it loosely as a raft of emotional problems that they say women suffer after having an abortion—nightmares, feelings of guilt, even suicidal tendencies—and compare it to post-traumatic stress disorder.[8]

The stresses associated with abortion are dismissed by *Ms. Magazine* as "a bogus affliction invented by the religious right." Grossman goes on to ask why campus therapists dealing with psychological problems don't ask women about whether they had an abortion. Her answer: "Because it's not politically correct. Campus counseling doesn't want to take the risk of suggesting that abortion can be traumatic—that's a word reserved for victims of rape, abuse, harassment, or natural disasters. So while everyone is bewildered at the mental health crisis on our campuses, not one voice suggests that perhaps the aftermath of abortion contributes to the staggering statistics."[9]

Imagine in this scientific age where investigations should be open, but "it's not politically correct" to ask a woman if her emotional problems can be related to an abortion. Why? Because if abortion advocates admit abortion can be traumatic, they would be contradicting their assertion that abortion-related psychological problems are rare.

6

Men Won't Buy the Cow

There are men who would rather cohabit with a woman and get free sex rather than get married. It's cheaper and safer than going to a prostitute. If he gets her pregnant, he'll insist on an abortion. Otherwise, he'll leave. A baby affects the money he earns, but it has no affect on his body. For him, an abortion is a simple solution that frees him from paying child support. When his sexual interest with her declines, he'll seek another woman. The first woman may end up being heart sick and broken, but he'll be happily on his way.

Who's the loser? Foolish women who comply. Women long for true love, affection, intimacy, and security. Some think by yielding their bodies they can build a lasting relationship, but this kind of man is just looking for someone to fulfill his sexual urges. Many only dig themselves deeper into a pit of discouragement and despair. Chuck Colson in *Breakpoint*, "For Better or Worse…Mostly Worse," tells this story:

> Tina wants to get married, but her boyfriend Ted just wants to move in. Ted is an exceptionally honest young man, so here is what he says: "Tina, I'm fond of you, and I want to live with you for the following reasons. First, it will make it easier for me to enjoy regular sex. Second, I want to protect my assets—assets I'd have to share with you if we got a divorce. Third, you already have kids, and I don't want to support them. Fourth, I'm waiting for my perfect soul mate to come along. Until I meet her, I'd like to live with you."

Sound convincing? Probably not. Tim's arguments are incredibly insulting. And yet, according to a new study, these are exactly the reasons men want to live with women—reasons that not only insult women, but also make them big losers on the domestic front.

At Rutgers University, researchers with the National Marriage Project have published a report called "Why Men Won't Commit: Exploring Young Men's Attitudes about Sex, Dating, and Marriage." The study offers the top ten reasons men are reluctant to say, "I do." Among them: They can get all the sex they want without marriage. They want to enjoy the single life as long as possible. They want to avoid the financial pitfalls of divorce. And they're afraid marriage will demand too many changes and compromises. Apparently, their live-in girlfriends can get used to their bad habits or leave.

Most galling of all is the admission by men that they don't want to marry their girlfriends because they're waiting for their "true love" to come along. Then they'll tie the knot, buy a home, and father kids. Meanwhile, their live-ins can pick up their socks and provide sex-on-demand.

Grandma was right: Men won't buy the cow if they can get the milk free....I hope this report serves as a wake-up call to women who think men who want to cohabit have marriage on their minds. Most of them do not.[1]

Limiting Your Partners

"Safe" sex advocates limiting your partners, preferably to one who is having sex with only you. So what do many men do? They find a temporary girlfriend to fulfill their sexual desires while they continue searching for "Miss Right." The frustrated girlfriend seeks a loving relationship while the boyfriend seeks only a sexual relationship.

Men aren't dummies. In order to get what they want, some tell their girlfriends what they want to hear. "I love you. One day I hope we'll get married. You're my dream come true." These men will insist their girlfriends take preventative measures like taking birth control pills so they can experience maximum sexual pleasure without the hazard of pregnancy.

Living Together

Janice Shaw Crouse, Ph.D., in "The Myths and Reality of Living Together Without Marriage," writes, "A college professor described a survey that he conducted over a period of years in his marriage classes. He asked guys who were living with a girl, point blank, 'Are you going to marry the girl that you're living with?' The overwhelming response, he reports, was 'NO!' When he asked the girls if they were going to marry the guy they were living with, their response was, 'Oh, yes; we love each other and we are learning how to be together.'"[2]

Crouse also reports, "In the United States, living together instead of marrying has become the norm for couples—half of young adults aged 20-40 are cohabiting instead of getting married. Cohabitation has increased nearly 1,000 percent since 1980, and the marriage rate has dropped more than 40 percent since 1960."

Why Living Together Is Popular

Why is living together without marriage so popular? "Safe" sex is taught in many schools across our nation. One of their popular messages for boys and girls is to "Be Faithful"—limit your sexual activity to only one partner who is having sex only with you. So what are many youth doing? They're cohabiting.

Some do it to get free sex; others think by living together they can test whether they are right for each other. That way when they do get married they will ensure a better marriage. However, Crouse reveals: "The divorce rates of women who cohabit are nearly 80 percent higher than those who do not. In fact, studies indicate that cohabiting couples have lower marital quality and increased risk of divorce." In conclusion Crouse writes, "A mass of sociological evidence shows that cohabitation is an inferior alternative to the married, intact, two-parent, husband-and-wife family. Increasingly, the myths of living together without marriage are like a mirror shattered by the force of the facts that expose the reality of cohabitation."[3]

Psychology Today in the article, "Living Together: More Popular, Still Risky," also reports: "Even though half of all couples live together before marriage, some Penn State researchers aren't so sure it is a good idea. They found that cohabitation before the ring is linked to troubled relationships and a higher rate of divorce."[4]

7

Pornography

Is viewing pornography just harmless fun? Are those opposed to pornography just old fashioned prudes? Some argue that pornography doesn't influence people. Then why is sex used so much by the advertising industry? What we see does affect our behavior. Listen to these teenagers:

> One day I was hanging out with a friend when I was 12. My friend showed me some pictures. I looked up websites and things would pop up and lead to other sites. It led me to having sexual intercourse at age 13, trying to do what I saw on the Internet. I got into drugs and wound up at House of Hope, a home for hurting teens.[1]

Here's another testimony from 16-year-old Bobby:

> When I was 11 years old I was on AOL and stuff started popping up. I said, "Oh, wow!! What's this?" Oh, I never saw anything like this and my curiosity caused me to go deeper and deeper. I downloaded pornographic pictures and then I started putting into practice some of the weird things I saw.[2]

Donna Rice Hughes in *Kids Online: Protecting Your Children in Cyberspace*, reported: "In a study of convicted child molesters, 77 percent of those who molested boys and 87 percent of those who molested girls admitted to the habitual use of pornography in the commission of their crimes."[3]

Deception of Pornography

Pornography is built on lies. It doesn't portray the real world of human sexuality. Pornography portrays women as hungry sex machines willing to accommodate men's sexual fantasies. This deception of the dehumanization of females leads to many social evils. The *Canadian Institute for Education on Family* reports:

> Canadian society has become an increasingly pornographic society in recent decades with disturbing implications for the children raised in it. Numerous scientific studies have demonstrated a strong correlation between exposure to pornography and subsequent deviant sexual behavior by children. The explosive growth of the Internet over the last decade and the freely available pornography to be found on this new medium pose an additional significant public health and safety threat to children….

> US study of teenagers exposed to "Hard core" pornography, "Two-thirds of the males and 40% of the females reported wanting to try out some of the behaviors they had witnessed. And, 31% of males and 18% of the females admitted doing some of the things sexually they had seen in the pornography *within a few*

days after exposure.".…

[And a] study found, "Exposure to sexually stimulating materials may elicit aggressive behavior in youth who are predisposed to aggression. Sexually violent and degrading material elicits greater rates of aggression and may negatively affect male attitudes toward women."[4]

Internet Porn

Wired stated in the article, "Internet Porn: Worse Than Crack?" that "Internet pornography is the new crack cocaine, leading to addiction, misogyny, pedophilia, boob jobs and erectile dysfunction, according to clinicians and researchers testifying before a Senate committee." Then it stated:

Witnesses before the Senate Commerce Committee's Science, Technology and Space Subcommittee spared no superlative in their description of the negative effects of pornography.

Mary Anne Layden, co-director of the Sexual Trauma and Psychopathology Program at the University of Pennsylvania's Center for Cognitive Therapy, called porn the "most concerning thing to psychological health that I know of existing today."

"The internet is a perfect drug delivery system because you are anonymous, aroused and have role models for these behaviors," Layden said. "To have drug pumped into your house 24/7, free, and children know how to use it better than grown-ups know how to use it—it's a perfect delivery system if we want to have a whole generation of young addicts who will never have the drug out of their mind."

Pornography addicts have a more difficult time recovering from their addiction than cocaine addicts, since coke users can get the drug out of their system, but pornographic images stay in the brain forever, Layden said. [5]

Beware! Don't get hooked on pornography! Avoid sexually active friends. The Internet makes it extremely easy to get access to porn. Many get addicted to it. The key—Flee from it; never get started. If you're addicted, get help. Pornography has destroyed many marriages and families. Some men are so addicted that they'll risk their jobs surfing the Web for pornography. Remember, pornography is built on lies. Don't feed your mind on this unrealistic fantasy that can destroy your future.

Memories and Depression

Those engaging in pornography and recreational sex retain memories of their sexual experiences. A premarital sex experience is like putting a red hot branding iron on the brain. This is what a 33 year-old woman said, "The hardest breakup I ever had was with the first person I had sex with. Fifteen years later, I still don't think I'm over him. I still dream about him and think about him and compare every guy since then to him. I'm married now and I feel like it's a threesome in my heart. He is still here. It is like he is a part of me and I still can't get over him."[6]

Who would want to marry a man addicted to pornography? Who would want to marry a woman who has had sex with all sorts of men, and who would want to marry a man who has had sex with numerous women? Everyone wants to marry a virgin. Why not become that person and present your future mate with a pure body?

Even if premarital sex was totally risk-free, it would still be unwise. Some think that once a sex act is done, it's finished. But it's not finished. The emotional bonding that took place and is now broken causes many to feel abused, violated, and depressed. A Heritage Foundation article states:

> When compared to teens who are not sexually active, teenage boys and girls who are sexually active are significantly less likely to be happy and more likely to feel depressed.
>
> When compared to teens who are not sexually active, teenage boys and girls who are sexually active are significantly more likely to attempt suicide.
>
> Thus, in addition to its role in promoting teen pregnancy and the current epidemic of STDs, early

sexual activity is a substantial factor in undermining the emotional well-being of American teenagers.[7]

U.S. News & World Report in "Risky Business," states:

Then there are the teens—and preteens—too young to fathom the consequences, both emotional and physical, of their behavior. Lynn Ponton, a professor of psychiatry at the University of California-San Francisco and author of *The Sex Lives of Teenagers*, says that this early initiation into sexual behaviors is taking a toll on teens' mental health. The result, she says, can be "dependency on boyfriends and girlfriends, serious depression around breakups and cheating, lack of goals—all of these things at such young ages."[8]

Warning!
Don't Let Your Mind Be Poisoned with Pornography

8

Myths and Truths

There are many fallacies about sex. Let's examine some of the myths and the truths about sex.

1. Myth: STDs can be effectively treated with antibiotics.

Truth: Antibiotic resistance is increasing. Some infections can be cured; others may appear cured but create future complications. Some STDs are incurable and will be with you until you die. For the rest of your life you could be taking medicine trying to stay healthy.

2. Myth: You can always tell if someone is infected with an STD.

Truth: Many STDs show no external symptoms.

3. Myth: You're cured once the symptoms of an STD go away.

Truth: Some symptoms go away even though the infection remains. Symptoms may reappear in the future and create serious complications.

4. Myth: Condoms protect you from STDs.

Truth: Condoms offer risk reduction for STDs, not total protection. Sometimes condoms fail.

5. Myth: Birth control pills protect you.

Truth: They may protect you from pregnancy, but offer no protection from STDs. They also fail.

6. Myth: You're not a man until you have sex.

Truth: It takes more manpower to abstain from sex than to yield to one's passions.

7. Myth: You're missing all the fun by abstaining from sex. We're having a blast with our boyfriends, partying, dancing, drinking, and having intimate relations.

Truth: I may be missing some temporary fun, but I'll have a much brighter future because I made a vow of abstinence till marriage. Besides, sex doesn't equal love, but sex can produce babies, STDs, depression, loneliness, despair, heartaches, loss of self-esteem, and a ruined reputation. I'm saving myself for my true lover on the day I get married.

Clean Girls

I was in the United States Marine Corp during the Korean War. After training I went to Camp Pendleton in southern California. Since I was from New York City, I decided to take a trip to a foreign country, Mexico. As I walked the streets of the border town of Tijuana, some taxicab drivers asked me, "Do you want a clean girl?"

Was I foolish enough to believe these drivers could provide a "clean girl"? They were out to make a buck. I wasn't the least bit interested. Some street girls are just painted sewers. They may be attractive, but who knows how many infectious diseases they carry?

Being Popular

Some of those loose girls are not walking the streets, but walking in school halls. They think having premarital sex will bring them ultimate feelings of love and fulfillment. They're dead wrong. Some yield to peer pressure to engage in sex so they'll be popular. In one survey, hundreds of sixth-to-ninth-graders were asked why they were having sex. Over 75 percent said to "fit in or to be cool." Only one student said, "Because I'm in love."

Loose girls may feel they're cool and popular, but many boys will look at them as promiscuous, slutty, and easy. Many of these girls will end up in despair because no self-respecting fellow will be interested in such a girl for marriage.

The Sexually Liberated

Some of the sexually active are proud and freely talk about their sexual encounters and their failed love affairs. Today's culture has resulted in many women becoming sexually coarsened and aggressive. These so called "sexually liberated women" are unashamed of their sexual exploits and freely discuss them. They ridicule virgins and consider themselves hip and cool.

Some sexually liberated women talk on TV about their ex's (ex-husbands) as if nothing happened. Don't believe it. Hidden behind their beautiful smiles are agonizing tears and heartaches from their search for lasting love and the man of their dreams. It's time for those who believe in abstinence from all sexual activities until marriage to stand up for their convictions and not be ashamed or intimidated.

Self-Esteem

Today's culture gives the impression that sexual attractiveness is the key to a woman's self-esteem. Many stores prominently display top-selling magazines with provocative covers that urge women to attract men with shocking attire and sexual techniques. Today, many women have also become addicted to pornography. Since sex is so body-focused, women often become dissatisfied with their bodies. Some diet even though they're not overweight; others have breast augmentation and cosmetic surgery to reach culture's unrealistic ideals.

Wise men and women learn to accept their bodies and focus instead on character issues like integrity, kindness, compassion, generosity, and courtesy. I'm not suggesting men and women shouldn't take care of themselves physically, but an obsession for a perfectly sculptured body instead of personality and character is unwise and unhealthy. Remember, many quality men are searching for women whose focus is on inner beauty rather than just on their looks.

Evolutionary Theory and Modern Science

Joe S. McIlhaney, obstetrician-gynecologist and founder/chairman of the Medical Institute for Sexual Health, and Freda McKissic Bush, obstetrician-gynecologist for over 20 years have coauthored the book, *Hooked*. They report, "We are drawn to the conclusion that modern evolutionary theory about human sexuality is wrong. This theory can be summarized by saying that those who propose it believe that human beings are (their terms) "designed" to be promiscuous."[1]

They state: "With the aid of modern neuroscience and a wealth of research, it is evident that humans are the healthiest and happiest when they engage in sex only with the one who is their mate for a lifetime."[2]

9

Solutions

W e've examined the many dangers of premarital sex, and they're scary. There's a very simple solution that will guarantee you'll never get a sexually transmitted disease: you and your spouse abstaining from sex until marriage. I want to stress that abstinence doesn't mean abstaining from sex forever; it means waiting for the time when true love can be expressed in a marriage union between a man and woman where ultimate sexual satisfaction can be realized.

Sex-Saturated Culture

Fulfilling this vow in our sex-saturated culture isn't easy. We're bombarded by print and video advertisers showing men and women embracing each other and glowing in ecstasy. They portray an artificial world. What they don't show you are the heartaches and devastating diseases that result from such freewheeling lifestyles. You need to be vigilant in your pursuit of purity because our culture over-emphasizes the body and sexual freedom apart from marital relations. Don't believe the lie that sexual liberation brings freedom.

When I grew up, girls guarded themselves from the passion of boys. Now, with educators teaching boys and girls that it's okay to engage in casual sex so long as proper precautions are employed, we have a rampant increase in sexually transmitted diseases. To stop this explosion of STDs and the associated heartaches and suffering, educators, parents, and youth need to firmly reject casual sex. Parents need to get into the driver's seat and teach the values that will teach their children how to become successful, rather than let today's sex-saturated culture dictate their children's future.

"But we live in a new age." We certainly do. But that's no excuse to follow the crowd. We need young people with backbones who will stand up and say, "Don't count me in when it comes to casual sex. My future is too important to be sacrificed for temporary pleasure."

Don't mistake infatuation for love. You may feel like you're walking on clouds and the sun is shining full force on your life—but when thunderstorms arise, your dreams will be shattered. True love will take you through storms. Infatuation is fleeting emotional love. Sadly, many youth make choices because of infatuation and suffer bitter consequences for their decisions.

The intelligent and simple solution: NO SEX UNTIL MARRIAGE! Sounds too simplistic? It's the solution that will guarantee you'll never pass on syphilis, genital warts, chlamydia, genital herpes, gonorrhea, trichomoniasis, or HIV/AIDS to your future marriage partner.

Sexual Abstinence Till Marriage

There is one, and only one, sound policy that provides guaranteed immunity from sexually transmitted diseases: Sexual abstinence until marriage for each marital partner. If humankind would adopt this policy, we'd see a screeching halt to the epidemic of STDs.

Many mock this. They claim that young people are undisciplined and will engage in sex. They promote recreational sex, and then wonder why millions of young people are infected every year with STDs. What's their solution? More sex education.

To prevent pregnancies sex educators do describe abstinence, the 100% effective method; but then they provide detailed descriptions about the pill, ring, shot, and patch to prevent ovulation; rhythm method which stresses abstinence during fertile days; spermicides to kill the sperm in the form of foam, jelly, suppository, or cream; barrier devices to stop the sperm such as diaphragm, sponge, cervical cap, and female and male condoms.

Now children are educated about sex. So what do many do? They use their new education to engage in various "safe" sexual activities. But many of these devices are totally useless in protecting against STDs. What happens? The statistics prove that many end up joining the ranks of those with STDs.

One wonders why educators provide detailed information about various methods to prevent pregnancies to young people in their formative years when some of these methods are ineffective in STD prevention. What does abstinence do? It encourages youth to control their bodies. How much heartache would be avoided if young people would take a strong stand for a life of abstinence till marriage?

How to Say, "NO!"

Youth face many sexual temptations. Here are helps and guidelines on how to say, "No!"

1. Be firmly committed to "No sex until marriage!"

2. Avoid attire and body language that encourages sexual responses. Dress for respect, not for arousal. Your dress should reflect the beauty of your personality and purity.

3. Abstain from looking at pornography on the Web and in magazines, reading sexually-stimulating novels, listening to degrading songs, and viewing movies and TV programs promoting immorality.

4. Don't ever let anyone touch the private parts of your body. Have a high level of self-respect.

5. Beware of the temptation when feeling lonely and depressed to yield to a sexual experience to find love. Hearing words like "I love you" might seem the answer to your dreams, but it isn't. Unscrupulous men often use these words to get what they want.

6. If you're in a relationship with someone who demands sex, immediately take the painful step and end the relationship. Set higher standards for your relationships, accepting only a person of character who'll honor and respect you, and not use you.

7. Remember, no condom protects the heart from guilt and depression. Live a life without guilt or regrets—choose a life of abstinence till marriage.

8. Be bold and let your commitment be known.

9. Avoid sexually active groups.

10. If you want a man or woman of high standards, find out where they meet and join them. Aim to associate with like-minded individuals. If you hang around where the "bad boys and girls" hang out, what can you expect? You may have a one-night exciting experience, but there's a good chance it will leave you depressed and lonely.

11. Avoid tempting situations like parties where alcohol and drugs are present.

12. Be mature enough not to feel lonely and left out when others participate in their sex-obsessed activities. Just wait. One day you'll hear their horror stories.

13. Find a friend who shares your commitment and encourage and support each other.

14. Consider your virginity as a gift. Save it for the one who will one day say, "I take you to be my wife," or "I take you to be my husband."

Unrealistic?

Is this unrealistic for today's culture? Absolutely not! There are many youth who are intelligent and want bright, healthy futures. They refuse to subscribe to the "safe" sex message. This is what one girl had to say:

Hi! I'm 17 years old. I dated a guy I thought was "the love of my life" two years ago. He pressured me to have sex. I thought it was wrong, and I was afraid of getting pregnant. I refused. He broke up with me and started dating someone else. I was heart-broken. Six months after our breakup, I met "J." "J" respected me, and said he would also save sex for marriage. I can't tell you how happy we are. We're perfect for each other in every way! We hope to get married some day. I'm so happy I'm saving myself for marriage. I don't even remember "what's-his name" now.[1]

Romantic emotions are extremely powerful, and it's easy to become physical. Be firm. Set definite limits to your physical relationship. If your partner pressures you, then you have a good indication this individual is selfish and doesn't respect you. Why go with someone who disrespects you? It will be extremely painful, but you'll be wise to end the relationship. You'll save yourself much heartache. Refuse to compromise your standards.

I will share some answers for dumb come-ons for casual sex. If you take a firm stand, you'll never need to use them.

Answers for Dumb Come-Ons

- I promise nothing will happen. (You can't tell what will happen.)
- If you love me, you'll let me. (If you really love me, you'll respect my wishes.)
- Everyone's doing it. (That's untrue. Besides, I don't care what others are doing, I'm not!)
- You've got to fit in. (If you have to have sex to fit in, call me, "Left out!" I don't want your company.)
- Watch this with me. (If it's promoting illicit sex in

movies, TV, or music, count me out. I refuse to let my mind become a garbage dump.)

• No one will find out. (They will if I get pregnant or get an STD.)

• I'll go only as far as you let me. (Stop now. I don't play with fire.)

• We're getting married; why wait? (We're not married, and until we are, it's NO!)

• Sex is no big deal. (That's what you think. Outside of marriage it can lead to a lifetime of disaster.)

• Oral sex is not sex. (Who are you kidding? Oral sex deals with sexual organs, so it's sex. Besides, STDs may be transmitted through oral sex.)

• Be popular. (So I can be known as the easy target?)

• Try it, you'll love it. (Yes I will—with the person I marry.)

• I'll use protection. (I don't believe in taking chances.)

• Trust me, I'm clean. (I know I am, and I'm staying that way!)

• You're the only virgin. (If I am, I'm proud of it!)

• I spent a lot of money on you. (What? Do you think I'm for sale?)

• You don't know what you're missing. (You think I'm stupid? I do know! I'll miss STDs, fear of pregnancy, guilt, and a host of emotional and psychological problems.)

Parents

Bernadine Healy, M.D. is the health editor for *U.S News and World Report* and writes its "On Health" column. She is a member of the President's Council of Advisors on Science and Technology, has served as the director of the National Institutes of Health, and is the president and CEO of the American Red Cross. In the article, "Let's Teach Our Children Well," Healy writes:

HELPING OUR KIDS DEVELOP INTO smart, tender, sexual beings is vital to their future happiness and as challenging as parenting gets. The perplexity of sex is that it's so compelling, such a power for good—and yet so dangerous for young people if they set off on the wrong track. Sex education in schools is beset with endless debate about abstinence only versus safe sex. What's missing and sorely needed is a focus on love and ennobling sexual intimacy as immutable currents in human life. Both as doctor and mother, I can't help but believe that our anything-goes society, in which impulses are immediately satisfied and sex is divorced from love and bonding, is simply not healthy physically, emotionally, or spiritually. [Caps in original.]

If we look at what today's teens are doing, it is enough to make parents weep and safe-sex educators recognize a need greater than condoms.[2]

This mother and doctor is greatly concerned of the free-wheeling sexual activities that today's youth are exposed to and are imitating. Healy says, "Young people account for half of the 19 million new STD cases each year." In comparison to adults, she states, "A teen, with an immature cervix, is more likely to catch an STD, triggering problems like smoldering pelvic inflammatory disease that can silently take away fertility, tubal pregnancies, cervical and even throat cancer, and transmission of disease to offspring at birth."

Then Dr. Healy says something that many kids hate to hear. "Parents are here to help their kids, each with his or her unique temperament, fulfill their dreams. And dreams of enduring love, encouraged, prepared for, and taken seriously, prompt wiser choices in general and nourish qualities like empathy, sincerity, and human closeness. It's not all sex talk; it's serious life talk, though it comes with the frustration of not quite knowing if—hello—anyone is listening."[3]

Is anyone listening? Let me ask you, when your parents speak to you, are you listening? Or are you like many who are so wise they don't need any advice? Unfortunately, today we're living in a culture that makes it cool to snap back and sass their parents. Many of these so-called "wise" teens will suffer tremendously because they refuse to listen to sound parental advice. I speak as a parent and one who has taught and observed teens for many years. You'll avoid many problems in life if you learn to trust and listen to your parents.

We parents were once just like you. We're willing to risk your wrath and tell you things you hate to hear. Why do we do this? It's not because we hate you or want to rule your life; we want you to have a happy and a successful future. We know that one of the quickest ways to destroy your future is to hang around wrong friends, spend time on the Internet at pornographic sites, go to drinking parties, engage in premarital sex, and do other harmful activities.

"But everyone is doing it."

"If in your crowd of friends everyone is doing it, you're in the wrong crowd. Find new friends where everyone is not doing it."

"It's so much fun."

"Racing down the highway going 100 mph is also fun. But you may hit an embankment and may live the rest of your life in a wheelchair."

Unfortunately, many teens are cocky and take pride in their wisdom. They refuse any correction. They're Mr. and Ms. Know-It-All. Their parents' hearts are broken over their defiance. But they couldn't care less. Let me warn you teens—you'll pay the price for your defiance. Some of you will never learn, and you'll suffer your entire life for your bitter and defiant attitude.

We're not perfect as parents, but along the way we've learned much. We love our kids and want the best for them. We could be permissive and let you do whatever you want and get you off our backs, but we know it will destroy your life. So we're willing for you to be angry with us. We'll lay down restrictions you hate. But one day when you're older, you'll look back and thank us for refusing to listen to you.

But some of you, in spite of your parent's best efforts, will defy your parent's instruction and hang around with friends your parents disapprove, will go to drinking parties, search the Internet for pornographic sites, and engage in premarital sex. Some of you because of your stubbornness and pride, and refusal to listen will end up singing the "Would've, Could've, Should've Blues."

Singing the "Would've, Could've, Should've Blues"

I would've never gotten an incurable STD, if I could've had different friends. But I should've said a bold, "NO!" instead of yielding to my boyfriend.

I would've been a virgin, if I could've avoided my first drink. I should've insisted that I don't drink.

I would've never lost my reputation, if I could've stood up for what I was taught. I should've done what I knew was right.

I would've never had gonorrhea of the throat, if I could've said, "No!" to oral sex. I should've ditched my boyfriend.

I would've never gotten pregnant, if I could've resisted peer pressure. I should've pushed him out of my life when he insisted on having sex.

I would've never been addicted to porn, if I could've avoided staring at those web pictures. I should've quickly left that first porn website.

Many youth, and many adults, also wish, "If I could only go back in life and do things over." Wishing to go back is a wasted dream. You can only move forward, never backward. You're young, so you can wish looking ahead. Wish yourself a bright future by vowing to abstain from all sexual activity until you're married. Then you won't be singing the "Would've, Could've, Should've Blues."

Dr. Bernadine Healy in the end of the article on "Let's Teach Our Children Well," tells what happened to her. "This past spring, I opened a Mother's Day card from our 28-year-old, just married daughter, embossed with just three words: 'You were right.' Music to any mom's heart."[4]

10

Rebel Virgins

What should you do about this onslaught of sexual pressures? Stand up and be assertive in your beliefs. Become a rebel virgin and refuse to let the sex activists intimidate you into silence.

Take even a stronger stance. When confronted with the "safe sex" message, respond, "Are you crazy? Do you think I want to jeopardize my future? Even if sex is 100% safe, I know it's not safe because of what it does to my mind and my future relations with my mate. I'm saving myself for a happy future."

State your boundaries boldly and dismiss the advice of those advocating casual sex; you'll save yourself much heartache. Remember, all major religions consider casual sex as wrong or sin. This belief is a strong motivation to abstain from premarital sex. Don't sacrifice your faith for temporary pleasure.

If you're going to college, be selective where you go. Refuse to go into dorms where men and women live together, for many of these dorms are like brothels. When you first arrive at college, make it a top priority to find groups that share your beliefs. Supportive groups are a great asset to help you remain true to your values.

Proud Virgins

Youth should realize that not everyone in college practices casual sex. There are groups of college students who are rebelling over the "hookup" culture and are proud about their virginity. MSNBC reported what two Harvard University seniors did to promote abstinence:

> Sometime between the founding of a student-run porn magazine and the day the campus health center advertised "Free Lube," Harvard University seniors Sarah Kinsella and Justin Murray decided to fight back against what they see as too much mindless sex at the Ivy League school.
>
> They founded a student group called True Love Revolution to promote abstinence on campus. The group, created earlier this school year, has more than 90 members on its Facebook.com page and drew about half that many to an ice cream social.[1]

The *New York Times* in "Students of Virginity," gave this report about Justin Murray, one-club founder of the Harvard group:

> "We found a huge body of scholarship that suggested conclusions that nobody on our campus was making," he says. They posted the conclusions on their Web site — the belief that " 'safe sex' is not safe"; that even the most effective methods of birth control can fail; that early sexual activity is strongly associated with all manner of terrible outcomes, from increased risk of depression to greater likelihood of marital infidelity, divorce and

maternal poverty. Premarital abstinence, on the other hand, is held up by True Love Revolution as improving health, promoting better relationships and, best of all, enabling "better sex in your future marriage."[2]

At Arizona State University, a group of students started a club, "The New Sexual Revolution," advocating the benefits of abstinence.

ASU New Sexual Revolution is a new, non-sectarian student organization dedicated to promoting discussion about the meaning and purpose of sexuality, the benefits of premarital sexual abstinence, the ethics and consequences of modern sexual exploitation, and the place of marriage and family life in society. The New Sexual Revolution looks to what current medicine, psychology, sociology, philosophy, and human experience teach us work toward the health and happiness both of the individual and of society. We also reflect on the sexual revolution of the 1960's and ask important questions: *Are we happier? Are we healthier? Where do we go from here?*" We seek to offer an alternative viewpoint to our peers on campus and in the larger community concerning such issues, and we welcome dissenting opinions, as we always strive toward informed, educated opinions and positions. We hope to offer support to those students on campus who have embraced abstinence and are looking for like-minded peers.[3]

Miss America Boldly Declaring Her Beliefs

Erika Harold was honored to be selected for the top 40 college student leaders in the nation by USA Today's All USA College Academic Second Team. She graduated from University of Illinois a Phi Beta Kappa and was accepted into Harvard University Law School. But instead of going to Harvard in the fall, Harold won the Miss America contest and would be spending a year touring the nation promoting the pageant's official platform, "Preventing Youth Violence and Bullying."

Before becoming Miss America, Erika Harold travelled and gave speeches encouraging teenagers to avoid premarital sex. To her, it was an important message. Now winning the title of Miss America, Harold felt this was a golden opportunity to continue to spread the message of abstinence from sex until marriage. However, she encountered a problem. The official platform for Miss America did not permit the message of abstinence from premarital sex. The Black Collegian Online writing about this event reports:

> Standing up to prevent youth violence is not a new endeavor for Harold, she committed to eradicating it long before becoming Miss America. She twice received the Miss America Organization's State Community Service Award for her platform, Teenage Sexual Abstinence: "Respect Yourself, Protect Yourself." And, for more than three years, she served as representative for Project

Reality, a national abstinence-centered education program, by discussing her views on the benefits of abstinence at national and state conferences, on radio programs, with legislative offices and in a written Congressional testimony.

She also spoke to thousands of students, organized countless events and designed informational handouts to encourage young people to construct and speak out about their own reasons for making a commitment to abstinence.

So, can you imagine her reaction when, after overcoming bullying in the ninth grade, being accepted into Harvard Law School, and finally having the chance to share her message with the nation's youth, she was "bullied" into not discussing sexual abstinence during her reign?

"One of my jobs as Miss America is to be a role model to young people and to provide them with my story as an example of how they can achieve positive things in their lives. My personal commitment to abstinence from drugs, sex and alcohol in my opinion helped me to accomplish many of my goals. If I were prevented from speaking about that I think it would be very disingenuous in terms of serving as a role model," said Harold, who plans to pursue a career in Public Interest Law and ultimately run for a public office.

"To suddenly become silent on this issue once I became Miss America would cause young people to whom I had already spoken to question where I stood on these issues and to question whether or not I still maintained my commitment."[4]

When Harold told the pageant officials that she wanted to speak about abstinence, they objected. It was a great honor to be elected Miss America, but Harold said, "I didn't want to waste the opportunity of being Miss America by not mentioning my commitment to abstinence."

To Harold, not being allowed to speak on a subject that was important to her was a waste of time being Miss America. If she couldn't speak about abstinence, then bullies would win.

"I will not be bullied,"[5] she told reporters when asked if she would avoid the subject. Harold spoke to the officials and explained saving sex is similar to avoiding drugs and alcohol. The pageant officials finally agreed she could include abstinence as part of her message.

CBS News had this to say about the incident:

There's nothing like a controversy over sex to get them worked up at the headquarters of the Miss America Pageant. The latest furor, though, has to do with NOT having sex.

Miss America Erika Harold is insisting on promoting abstinence during her yearlong reign, to the chagrin of the pageant. Conservatives have rallied to her cause and accused the pageant of hypocrisy, giving the Miss America organization the kind of clobbering it usually gets from the left.

"In an age where beauty queens are regularly disqualified for inappropriate behavior, who would have thought a virtuous one would be silenced for her virtue?" said Sandy Rios, president of conservative group Concerned Women for America....

Rios said the Miss America organization's stand "betrays a hidden agenda of political correctness and religious bigotry among pageant officials. They are attacking Erika Harold's values, which goes completely against what everyone thought the Miss America pageant stood for."

Bridget Maher, family policy analyst for the Family Research Council, said the pageant was undermining its own efforts to promote women in seeking to muzzle Harold's pro-abstinence views.

"By encouraging young people to abstain from sex until marriage, Miss America is teaching them not to view women as sex objects but to value them as people," Maher said.[6]

Sentiments of the Founders of Our Nation

Youth need to know the sentiments the founders of our nation had concerning religion and government. Congress unanimously passed the Northwest Ordinance on July 13, 1787. Its purpose was to establish a basic governing system for the Northwest Territory, which consisted of a huge amount of land extending from the Great Lakes to the Ohio River valley. The leaders of our nation stated in this ordinance, "There shall be neither slavery nor involuntary servitude in the said territory." It also said, "Religion, morality, and knowledge, being necessary to good government and the happiness of mankind, schools and the means of education shall forever be encouraged."

That was the sentiment of the early founders of our nation. Teddy Roosevelt said, "To educate a person in the mind but not in morals is to educate a menace to society." Religion and the founding of our nation is an important issue. If you want to learn more, go to www.advancepublishing.com and under "Free Resources" you may read the free book that I wrote: *Schools in Crisis: Training for Success or Failure?* It goes into much more detail.

But what's happening in many of our public schools? Religion, which is a strong advocate for sexual abstinence until marriage, is ridiculed. In this new culture of "anything goes" mentality, many young people lose their faith and throw off their moral restraints. Their earlier vows of abstinence until marriage, many taken in a religious environment, are often rejected.

In today's educational culture of tolerance, there's one area where it's culturally permissible to be intolerant—toward those expressing religious beliefs, especially Christian beliefs. A popular hypocritical method of rejecting arguments is to label the opponents' views as coming from the religious right. Opponents using these unreasonable tactics need to be exposed that they are the ones who are intolerant. Our nation needs youth who will explore the foundational beliefs that made our nation great and boldly promote those values.

Renewed Purity

What if you've made a mistake and engaged in premarital sex? It is never too late to renew your life and pursue purity. Living a life of purity is about your future. The past can't be changed, but the future can be. Set your sights on choosing a lifestyle so the person who becomes your future mate will respect you as a person of character.

Make a vow of renewed purity by stating, "I will never again engage in any sexual activity before marriage!" Now get back in the driver's seat and take control of your life. If you have emotional problems from premarital sex, seek a trusted, educated counselor who can help you solve your problems.

If your friends know you were sexually active, declare your new commitment boldly. If your friends are sexually active, search for new friends. Date only those who share your beliefs.

Psychiatrist Miriam Grossman emphasizes in her book, *Unprotected*, "The message must get out: casual sex is a health hazard for young women."[7] Grossman says:

> We *do* know that most women who have been infected discover it in a startling way—when they can't conceive. Since in up to 80 percent of infected women, chlamydia produces no pain, fever, or discharge, a woman thinks she's fine. Like her infected cells, she's an unsuspecting hostess to a dangerous guest. Years later, when she's settled down, married, and put the partying

and hookups behind her, she's told that her blood has antichlamydial antibodies—evidence of old infection. The doctor puts a scope through her navel to look at her fallopian tubes, and discovers they are enlarged and scarred by adhesions. And this is the reason she cannot have a baby.[8]

Pity the poor husbands and wives when they get this message that they will never be able to bring a child into the world. Imagine the guilt and heartaches the wives must have when they learn their infertility is caused by their youthful premarital sexual encounters.

Tips for a Happy Future

Here are tips for a happy and prosperous future:

1. Set clear standards and boundaries when dating. The goal of romance should be getting to know each other and having fun, not sexual intimacy. Avoid sexual temptations. Go on group dates. Save one-on-one dates for times when you're serious about marriage. Learn to have fun with groups.

2. Don't advertise your sexuality with your attire. Dress in a way that attracts the kind of person you desire. Aim to show less skin and skin tight clothes. Avoid being trashy and sexy; be feminine and ladylike. Let your inner beauty be your hallmark. There are many good men longing for women of that caliber.

Excellent character, as honesty, modesty, kindness, humility, friendliness, and willingness to listen, are more important than good looks for attracting high-quality men. Likewise for men, there are many noble women looking for men of character.

3. Obey your conscience: the moral code that tells you what's right and wrong.

4. Make decisions to build healthy relations. Don't pursue "I'm young only once." One bad decision can result in a lifetime of remorse.

5. A healthy relationship is built on mutual trust. An unhealthy relationship is exploitive and leaves you hurting and depressed.

6. If a boyfriend or girlfriend demands sex—he or she isn't a friend. Cut off the relationship, regardless how painful. You'll avoid many future problems.

7. Raise your dating standards and be selective. Avoid pornography and sexually active friends. Beware of dating those addicted to pornography. Their sexual fantasies may continue after marriage and be a road block to having a satisfying relationship.

8. If you associate with sexually active people, you'll be pressured to do the same. There are many faith-based organizations and groups that stress abstinence till marriage. Associate with friends who share your beliefs. Refuse to be embarrassed or intimidated by the sexually active.

9. As intelligent beings, we want to protect our

bodies. Why not include the mind and heart? Refuse to look at soft and hard-core pornography on cable, Internet, magazines, and videos. Avoid sexually suggestive music; television shows promoting sex, drugs and alcohol; tongue kissing; spending time alone in cars and the privacy of a bedroom; and allowing yourself to be fondled in your private areas. Filling minds with unrealistic sexual fantasies encourages sexual arousals. Don't let your mind and heart become a garbage dump.

10. Don't believe the TV ads and Hollywood scenes making the euphoria of love appear to last forever. Even in healthy, loving marriages, infatuation fades. When mates possess true love, they don't depend on their emotions. Their intimate love causes them to share their opinions, values, secrets, fears, joys, and sorrows. This love is also kind, considerate, unselfish, respectful, and sacrificial.

11. Learn to be happy with yourself. Don't let yourself believe that only another person can make you happy.

12. Build your dating on communication, not sex. One of the most important issues to having a happy marriage is communicating with one another and being a good listener. One of the major reasons for divorce is lack of communication. Seek a partner who desires to communicate with you and listens to your concerns. A marriage built only on physical attraction doesn't satisfy.

13. There are many good-looking women and handsome men who would make a disastrous spouse. What's important in marriage is character. So choose someone possessing character. One of the best indicators of a person's character and how they will treat you is how they treat their parents. If they're disrespectful to their parents, they'll be disrespectful to you. If they're loving and kind to their parents, it's much more likely you'll get the same treatment. Be alert. Another good source of information about the one you're dating is to ask your parents. They'll often give you the wisest and best evaluation.

14. Above all, be the kind of person you'd want to marry. Set your standards high by being respectful, hardworking, trustworthy, loyal, and pure. You may be teased because you're not dating much, but ignore the teasing. When you attract someone with like standards, you'll reap a lifetime of rewards.

A college student shared his experience of finding the girl of his dreams. "With her," he says, "there was never a dull moment. We totally clicked." But instead of strengthening their relationships with communicating, through his initiation they began having sex.

He then reports, "Sex soon became the focus of our relationship. I stopped wanting to get to know her on any other level. And so, instead of growing closer together, we actually started drifting apart...But when my girlfriend and I started relating mostly physically, it short-circuited the other parts of our relationship. As a result, the relationship as a whole started to go south. We might still be together today if we (I) had waited."[9]

This young man lost the girl of his dreams. The solution for a happy future with your sweetheart is to avoid sexual activity and concentrate on relationship building. Let's examine the benefits of sexual abstinence till marriage.

11

The Benefits

You're young now, but one day you'll probably want to get married. Would you want to marry someone who had numerous sexual relations? I was fortunate that my wife and I were virgins when we married. Did I have sexual temptations? Certainly. At the age of 21 I was drafted into the Marine Corps during the Korean War. For two years I served my country. Then I met my wife in church and dated her for 1 ½ years. Did I have sexual passions? You bet I did.

But what did we do? We're normal. Our sexual hormones were aroused, but we controlled the fire within us. We refused to do anything sexual. We were happy and had many fun times together. We discovered that we were deeply in love, and we decided to get engaged. We set our wedding date, got married, and finally fulfilled that ultimate longing for intimacy. What happened afterward is too personal to reveal, that sacred moment when two virgins have the right to fulfill their sexual desires.

Did I ever have to worry about contracting a sexually transmitted disease? Never. Why? Because both of us never engaged in premarital sex. I made a marriage vow that I'd be faithful to her, and to this day I've never broken that vow. We never had any fears of sexual diseases. Think of that statement. No fear of genital herpes, gonorrhea, HIV/AIDS, genital warts, syphilis, or a host of other STDs. Pity those who listened to the "safe" sex advocates that recreational sex is okay so long as proper precautions are used, but somehow, in the heat of passion, they contracted an STD.

Does that mean my wife and I don't encounter sexual temptations? Certainly we do. But since we were disciplined to be pure before marriage, we continue to reject all sexual temptations. Like many married couples, we encountered sickness, disagreements, and financial difficulties, but since we vowed to stay together until death do us part, we worked through them and continue to love and enjoy one another.

Children came along and witnessed happy parents still in love. They in turn found mates and became happily married. Today, we've been happily married for 53 years, and have five children and 19 grandchildren.

Traditional and Modern Wedding Vows

Unfortunately, today some have modernized the traditional wedding vow for a more personalized one. Now some are saying their wedding vow as: "For as long as we continue to love each other," or "For as long as our love shall last," or "Until our time together is over."

Is marriage reduced to staying together until either partner loses interest in another? Can you find true happiness in that kind of temporary commitment? Let's look at a traditional wedding vow for the man:

Will you love her, comfort her, honor and keep her, in sickness and in health, for richer, for poorer, for better, for worse, in sadness and in joy, to cherish and continually bestow upon her your heart's deepest devotion, forsaking all others, keep yourself only unto her as long as you both shall live?

When I got married, I made that vow for as long as we both shall live. We combined our bank accounts and all our belongings. That was 53 years ago. Regardless of what happens to my wife, I vowed I'll always be by her side. If she's sick and disabled, I'll be there for her. I've told my sweetheart numerous times, "Honey, regardless what happens, I'll always take care of you."

A number of years ago my wife had difficulty walking because of a problem with one of her knees. We had a cruise planned to Europe. I took a wheelchair along and wheeled her around. I limited myself because of her weakened condition. I wanted to make my wife happy.

Elizabeth Cohen of the CNN Medical Unit reports, "Terminally ill cancer patients have a higher-than-average divorce rate, and it's almost always the husband leaving his sick wife."[1] Imagine how that woman feels. How would you like it if you became sick, and the one you married said, "Remember, we made a vow, 'For as long as our love shall last.' Well, my love is gone, so I'm leaving." You'd be devastated.

My wife and I made a vow to remain together whether "for richer, for poorer, for better, for worse, in sadness and in joy." It took me ten years to write my first book, *Schools in Crisis: Training for Success or Failure?* I took a year's leave of absence from a teaching position as a high school teacher in New York

City to write that book. We have five children, and I used up all my savings when I was on this leave of absence. I told my wife not to purchase cake for dessert in order to save money. My wife never complained. She was willing to live a poorer lifestyle because of my vision to transform the educational system. Today, I own three businesses, and one of them is the largest of its kind west of the Mississippi River. It didn't matter to my wife whether we were rich or poor.

Forsaking All Others

There's another very important aspect of the traditional vow: "To cherish and continually bestow upon him your heart's deepest devotion, forsaking all others." That means there'll be no more love affairs with others. Will you be tempted once you're married? Absolutely! There are handsome men and gorgeous women that have no qualms about going with someone who is married. But we made a vow—FORSAKING ALL OTHERS!

An interesting incident happened to my wife and me. Our publishing company had a booth at the American Library Association in Washington, D.C. Since our hotel was near a park close to the White House, we decided to rest awhile by sitting on a bench under a flowering crepe myrtle. I had my arm around my wife, and we were holding hands. Two women came by. Seeing us being affectionate with each other, one of the women asked with tears in her eyes, "How long have you been married?"

"We've been married 52 years," I replied.

We talked awhile, and this woman told us that she hoped

she would have a marriage like ours. Her ten-year marriage was filled with difficulties.

Here we were, an old couple just simply in an unobtrusive way showing our affection for one another. Everyone longs to be loved; it's universal. My love for my wife is not a put on. We kiss each other when we get up in the morning, when one of us leaves the home, when we return, and when we go to bed. I often tell my wife I love her. Now don't laugh, but I still call my wife sweetie, honey, sweetheart, and babe. My goal in life is to make my wife happy. That's her goal, too, to make me happy. We're not perfect, but the ideal marriage is when both husband and wife constantly aim to make each other happy.

It's a paradox. If you aim only to make yourself happy you'll be miserable. Aim to make others happy and you'll find fulfillment and joy. Try it; you'll discover it works.

Often I introduce my wife as "my sweetheart." When I mention how long we're married, the response I often get is, "Don't hear of marriages lasting that long anymore."

Why not? Too many have swallowed the lies of our popular culture. Everyone wants a happy future, and most want their future to include a happy family. But today we're witnessing the breakdown of the family in America. But it doesn't have to be that way for you. You can have a happy marriage if you take the proper steps.

Wish

How many of you wish that on your wedding day you could give your lover-for-life the pure body of a virgin? Can you imagine the happy and unifying sexual experience when you marry and join together in a lifetime commitment to unity? This type of sexual unity is something much bigger than a temporary joyride; it's a loving, total commitment when two become one. Make this wish for sexual purity one of your highest priorities. Don't sacrifice your virginity for a temporary thrill that can lead to devastating results.

Devastated Marriages

However, think of those marriages where the husband and wife in their youth were flippant about their bodies and satisfied their lustful passions. If it felt good, they did it with numerous partners. They never mastered the art of building a nonsexual loving relationship. Instead, their sexual exploits sowed seeds of mutual distrust. The husband doesn't trust his wife, and the wife doesn't trust her husband.

What happens to those who followed the "safe" sex message when they get married and have never mastered resisting sexual temptations in their youth? Their sexual flame is short-lived, and many end up cheating and seeking extra marital partners. They forsake their vows of being faithful as long as they both shall live.

Their sexual exploits become discovered, and then the painful divorce process begins. But what you don't hear is the constant friction in the home before the divorce—the anger, yelling, accusations, depression, frustration, fears, tears, verbal and sometimes physical abuse, and anxiety. Their home becomes a perpetual battleground. After many arguments and fights over unfaithfulness, many get divorced. Some of these divorces involve children, and many children suffer because of living in this atmosphere of constant turmoil and accusations.

Cheating by a husband or wife is one of the major reasons for divorce. I'm not saying everyone unfaithful before marriage will be unfaithful after marriage. However, those who mastered a disciplined lifestyle of abstinence are far more likely to remain faithful after marriage and reap the many benefits of a happy and fruitful marriage.

There's much more about having a happy marriage, but making a permanent vow is an important first step. You can view the video, "Straight Talk" at www.advancepublishing. com under "Free Resources," where I share insight about sex, marriage, and a host of other relevant subjects.

Happy Future

We live in a culture that promotes sexual self-fulfillment. It's a false dream that leads many to a road of failure and despair instead of a happy future. The road to success and happiness is a road of self-discipline.

Abstinence till marriage is a life of self-discipline that suppresses sexual hormones and brings them under control. Abstinence brings freedom: freedom from comparisons of previous sexual encounters, freedom from all sexually transmitted diseases, and freedom to pursue a life of finding true love. Abstinence allows you to resist premature relationships so you can dedicate yourself to pursue your dreams. Abstinence is much more than just saying, "No," to sex. It's a choice that says, "One day I want a loving and enduring relationship that will lead to a happy and fulfilling marriage where sex can be enjoyed in its fullness."

It's difficult for youth to think that anything can eclipse sex. Everything around them screams this message of the joy of sex. But if you think marriage is all about sex, you're greatly mistaken. It's about having a loving relationship. Certainly sex is part of it, but only as it relates to a loving relationship. There's earning a living, shopping, cooking, children, financial decisions, taxes, careers, and many other decisions in keeping a happy home functioning.

Goals

What are your goals for one year, five years, and ten years? What actions can you take to prepare yourself for a great future? The many dangers of premarital sex can become a disastrous for your future in reaching your goals; whereas a life of abstinence for both you and the one you one day plan to marry can only result in benefits.

Abstinence till marriage is more than just protecting yourself from disease, pregnancy, and possible humiliation. It's preparing yourself for a wonderful relationship with a partner where you can experience the deepest level of untarnished love and intimacy.

Which will make you happier, healthier, and more successful—being active sexually or practicing abstinence till marriage? It's obvious. Is it difficult in this sex-saturated culture? Definitely! What's the solution for preparing the best future for yourself? The so solution if for *you* to join the new generation and challenge the sex-saturated culture.

A New Generation and the Challenge

Our nation needs a new generation of youth who are self-disciplined and unashamed of their virginity. When Erika Harold was chosen to be Miss America, she refused to be bullied into silence about the message of abstinence from sex until marriage. She said, "My personal commitment to abstinence from drugs, sex and alcohol in my opinion helped me to accomplish many of my goals. If I were prevented from speaking about that I think it would be very disingenuous in terms of serving as a role model."[2] She stood her ground and won permission to speak on the values of abstinence.

Like Erika, these bold and intelligent youth will refuse to risk their futures with untimely pregnancies, contracting sexually transmitted diseases, and the emotional baggage left from sexual encounters. They understand the many dangers not mentioned by the "safe" sex advocates and the many advantages of remaining virgins until marriage. They're more interested in making a better future for themselves than short-lived sexual adventures that may result in a lifetime of disasters.

These youth are neither intimidated nor deceived. They're able to pierce the smiley fraudulent mask of the sexually active and boldly challenge them. They'll expose the false claims of the evolutionary theory that states humans are designed for being promiscuous until they find the one with the best genes.

Instead, these intelligent youth will support scientific findings, who as Joe S. McIlhaney, obstetrician-gynecologist and founder/chairman of the Medical Institute for Sexual Health, and Freda McKissic Bush, obstetrician-gynecologist for over 20 years, have reported in their book, *Hooked: New Science on how Casual Sex is Affecting Our Children*: "Modern breakthroughs in neuroscience research techniques and this new data now accumulating are leading to a major change in approach to sexual behavior understanding and recommendations. The science says that generally speaking, the healthiest behavior, both physically and emotionally, is for persons to abstain from sex until they can commit to one partner for the rest of their life."[3]

These youth realize that giving their husband or wife their virgin body is one of the most priceless gifts they can provide on their wedding night. They have not yielded to their instincts, but have been disciplined. Now they'll reap the great reward of pure intimacy, free from any scarred memories, guilt, or remorse.

This new generation will stand up, put their shoulders back, and refuse to become discouraged or intimidated by the onslaughts of the entrenched bureaucracy of the "safe" sex advocates or by their favorite attack of labeling opponents as bigoted, religious, and intolerant. These brave youth are convinced that with abstinence as their standard for sexual behavior, they'll have much happier marriages, sex lives, children, and futures. In addition, they realize the future prosperity of our nation hinges on what this new generation will do.

Will You Proudly Join This New Generation?

12

The Vow

We need responsible youth who will boldly take the "Abstinence Till Marriage" (ATM) vow. I know you want a happy life. Everyone does. For your future success, I urge you to sign this vow. Make a firm commitment that from this day forward, you'll abstain from sex until the day you get married. Notice it must be a "firm commitment." It's one thing to make a vow, but when a sexually attractive person enters your life, it's very tempting to violate that vow.

Many make abstinence pledges in groups because everyone else is doing it, and they feel pressured by their parents. They're not really making a firm commitment for abstinence till marriage. They're crowd pleasers. In the emotional flames of sexual heat, many non-committed pledgers fail to restrain themselves. Opponents like to mention these failed abstinence pledgers when they promote their "safe" sex message. If you're not firmly committed, don't sign the ATM pledge.

Second Vow

Or perhaps this is you: "I've failed. I'm no longer a virgin. I'm devastated over my past."

Is there any hope? Definitely! We all make mistakes in life, some more serious than others. There's a simple solution. Recognize your mistakes and rebuild your self-esteem. Build the inner beauty of your character. Don't rely on the opposite sex for your approval. Vow to become a second virgin. Vow you'll never again allow anyone to pressure you into sex. Get a physical exam to make certain you don't have any STDs. Remember, some STDs show no physical signs.

Future Vow

If you plan on getting married one day, you'll be making another extremely important future vow. Would you want to make a wedding vow to one who has been sexually active, or one who like you had the self-discipline to be abstinent until marriage? There's no question that everyone would want to marry a virgin. This ATM vow will strongly reinforce your wedding vow and help you to have a happy future.

Benefits for Making a Vow to Save Sex for Marriage

Taking the vow to abstain from sex until marriage simplifies your life. Now you may concentrate on your goals without fear of untimely pregnancy or contracting STDs. List your goals for your life. Respect yourself and aim high.

Making this abstinence till marriage vow doesn't guarantee success. Peer pressure and sexual temptations are powerful. To counteract these pressures, you must be strong and courageous to stand up for the principles you believe in. Gather in places where quality people meet. Look for friends who share your values. Never let the momentary pleasure of sex ruin your life. Don't let those boasting about their sexual encounters intimidate you. Remember, the choices you make will determine your future and this nation's future. Here is a brief summary of benefits of saving sex for marriage.

Benefits When Both Partners Abstain from All Sexual Activities Till Marriage

1. Freedom from all STDs and their devastating complications

2. Freedom from fear of an untimely pregnancy

3. Not becoming a teen parent who often drops out of school and is on welfare, and whose children tend to have lower intelligence scores, are prone to fail in school, abuse drugs, and end up in prison

4. No financial obligations caused by an untimely child

5. No fear of becoming sterile because of an STD infection

6. Never fearing contracting HIV and ending up with AIDS

7. Freedom from the emotional hang-ups of guilt, doubt, disappointments, and fears from previous sexual relations

8. Not prone to the depression and suicide that sexually active youth encounter

9. A reputation for being trustworthy and respectful

10. Become more attractive to people of like character

11. Increased self-respect

12. Strengthens the ability to refuse other health-endangering behaviors, such as smoking, alcohol, and drugs

13. Produces positive effects by providing greater energy to pursue dreams

14. Avoids a tarnished reputation

15. Gives peace of mind

16. Provides greater capability to resist peer pressure

17. Helps build relationships on love and trust, not sex

18. Strengthens love and relationship building

19. Provides greater ability to have a strong, happy, and fulfilling marriage

20. Greatly improves your chances for a better home when children arrive

21. No fear of comparisons or false expectations and flashbacks from previous sexual encounters

22. Greater joy of intimacy when married

23. Being faithful before marriage helps to remain faithful after marriage

24. Better for your health

25. Allows you to pursue your hopes and dreams for a bright future

Abstinence Till Marriage Vow*

So for the sake of your health and for a bright future, I urge you to sign the ATM statement and pledge your commitment to sexual purity. This is also for those making a second pledge for sexual abstinence. Will you be disciplined and bold with your beliefs, believe in your dignity, and aim to associate with like-minded people? Then join the winner's club by signing the ATM pledge.

*Permission is granted to make copies of the vow on the following page. Also go to www.advancepublishing.com and under "free resources" you may print various formats of this vow.

Abstinence Till Marriage Vow

As of today, I choose to make a firm commitment for abstinence till marriage. In order to have a happy marriage, I vow to present to my future mate a pure body without the potential effects of sexual diseases and the emotional baggage from premarital sexual activities. I will endeavor to be bold and encourage others with similar values to fulfill their commitment.

I _____ pledge from this day on I will refrain from all sexual activities till marriage.

Signature _____

Date _____

My Reasons for Signing the Vow

_____

_____

_____

_____

_____

_____

_____

Notes

1. The Challenge

[1] http://www.leaderu.com/orgs/probe/docs/epid-std.html

[2] *The Associated Press*, March 12, 2008. (Forhan SE, Gottlieb SL, Sternberg MR, et al. Prevalence of sexually transmitted infections and bacterial vaginosis among female adolescents in the United States: data from the National Health and Nutrition Examination Survey 2003-2004. In: 2008 National STD Prevention Conference, Chicago, Illinois; March 10-13, 2008.)

[3] Grossman, M.D., Miriam, *Unprotected*, Sentinel, Published by Penguin Group, 2007.

[4] Ibid. p. 3.

[5] Ibid. pp. 1-6.

[6] Ibid. p. 4.

2. The Battle

3. The Dangers

[1] www.cdc.gov/std/HPV/STDFact-HPV.htm

[2] *Readers Digest,* "The Farther Shore," August, 2008.

[3] *Daily Mail*, "The true cost of sex under 16," December 8, 2007.

[4] http://www.ywwf.org, (Blount Nurses for Health Education), "Date Raped After Drinking Beer."

[5] http://www.hhs.gov/pharmacy/phpharm/hpstd.html

4. Sexually Transmitted Diseases

[1] *U.S. News & World Report*, "Risky Business," May 27, 2002.

[2] *U.S. News & World Report*, "Clueless About Risks of Oral Sex," March 10, 2008.

[3] www.smartersex.org/safe_sex/safe_sex.asp

[4] www.cdc.gov/STD/stats05/trends2005.htm

[5] *The Associated Press*, March 11, 2008. From http://www.msnbc.msn.com/id/23574940.

[6] *USA Today*, "Gonorrhea mutates to resist antibiotic treatment," April 13, 2007.

[7] http://www.avert.org/worldstats.htm

[8] http://www.cdc.gov/hiv/topics/msm/resources/factsheets/msm.htm

[9]"Lesbian, Gay, Bisexual and Transgender Health," http://www.cdc.gov/lgbthealth/

[10] *International Journal of Epidemiology*, Volume 26, pp. 657-661.

[11] *Houston Chronicle*, "A dark side to good news of living longer with HIV?" December 8, 2007.

[12] *Consumer Reports*, "Birth control More & safer choices," February 2005.

[13] Grossman, M.D., Miriam, *Unprotected*, Sentinel, Published by Penguin Group, 2007, pp. 29-30.

5. Pregnancy and Abortion

[1] www.ywwf.org, (Blount Nurses for Health Education), "Teenage Pregnancy Limits Present And Future Plans."

[2] http://www.time.com/time/magazine/article/0,9171,1074861-1,00.html

[3] Ibid.

[4] Grossman, M.D., Miriam, *Unprotected*, Sentinel, Published by Penguin Group, 2007, pp. 78-80.

[5] Ibid. p. 83.

[6] http://afterabortion.com/new_visitors.html

[7] Grossman, M.D., Miriam, *Unprotected*, Sentinel, Published by Penguin Group, 2007, p. 89.

[8] http://www.msmagazine.com/aug01/pas.html

[9] Grossman, M.D., Miriam, *Unprotected*, Sentinel, Published by Penguin Group, 2007, pp. 90-91.

6. Men Won't Buy the Cow

[1] http://www.breakpoint.org/listingarticle.asp?ID=5355 Breakpoint, "For Better Or Worse…Mostly Worse," July 24, 2002.

[2] http://www.crosswalk.com/marriage/11531429/

[3] Ibid.

[4] *Psychology Today*, "Living Together: More Popular, Still Risky," August 7, 2003.

7. Pornography

[1] http://www.protectkids.com/effects/teentestimonials.htm

[2] Ibid.

[3] Donna Rice Hughes, *Kids On Line: Protecting Your Children in Cyberspace*, Revell, 1988, comments taken from www.protectkids.com/effects/harms.htm

[4] http://www.cief.ca/research_reports/harm.htm

[5] http://www.wired.com/science/discoveries/news/2004/11/65772.

[6] McIlhaney, Joe S., Bush, Freda McKissic, *Hooked*, Northfield Publishing, Chicago, 2008, p. 111.

[7] http://www.heritage.org/Research/Abstinence/cda0304.cfm

[8] *U.S. News & World Report*, "Risky Business," May 27, 2002.

8. Fallacies and Truths

[1] McIlhaney, Joe S., Bush, Freda McKissic, *Hooked*, Northfield Publishing, Chicago, 2008, pp. 136-137.

[2] Ibid. p. 136.

9. Solutions

[1] http://www.ywwf.org, (Blount Nurses for Health Education), "Found Love From Someone Who Respects Her."

[2] *U.S. News & World Report*, "Let's Teach Our Children Well," September 27,2008.

[3] Ibid.

[4] Ibid.

10. Rebel Virgins

[1] http://www.msnbc.msn.com/id/17740428/ (From Associated Press, March 22, 2007.)

[2] *The New York Times*, "Students of Virginity," March 30, 2008.

[3] http://asu.edu/clubs/newsexualrevolution/aboutUs.htm

[4] http://www.black-collegian.com/issues/2ndsem03/america2003-2nd.shtml

[5] *Campus Life*, "Miss America's Unpopular Stand," March/April 2003

[6] http://www.cbsnews.com/stories/2002/11/15/entertainment/main529610.shtml

[7] Grossman, M.D., Miriam, *Unprotected*, Sentinel, Published by Penguin Group, 2007, p. 28.

[8] Ibid. p. 110.

[9] http://www.leaderu.com/everystudent/sex/articles/wolves.html

11. The Benefits

[1] http://archives.cnn.com/2001/HEALTH/05/14/cancer.divorce/index.html

[2] http://www.black-collegian.com/issues/2ndsem03/america2003-2nd.shtml

[3] McIlhaney, Joe S., Bush, Freda McKissic, *Hooked*, Northfield Publishing, Chicago, 2008, p. 136.

12. The Vow

Index

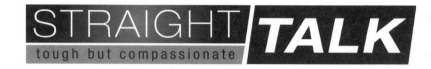

Free Online Videos

Straight Talk is hard-hitting, fast-paced, provocative, yet compassionate. Carl Sommer does not shy away from challenging issues as he offers from his vast experiences practical solutions to help students on their quest for success.

Sommer shares his insights on the dangers of drugs, alcohol, sex, and dating, and offers sound advice about friends, peer pressure, self-esteem, entering the job market, careers, entrepreneurship, the secrets of getting ahead, and much more.

To View Free Online Videos Go To:

www.AdvancePublishing.com

Under "Free Resources" click on "Straight Talk"

Teen Success In Career & Life Skills
If You Don't Want the Truth, Don't Read This!

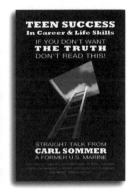

Carl Sommer's straight talk is used to help youth find their way in today's culture. From his vast experiences as a former U.S. Marine, high school teacher, assistant dean of boys, foreman, operations manager, and currently owner of three businesses and an award-winning author, Sommer shares many practical insights both from his experiences and a host of others many practical insights to help teens become successful both in school and in the workplace.

Explore

- The Challenge and Your Dream
- Educational Success or Failure
- The Technology Explosion
- Choosing and Preparing for Your Career
- The Resume, Interview, and Advancing On the Job
- Understanding the Free Enterprise System
- Elephant Ears, Eagle Eyes, and a Pinhole Mouth
- The Importance of Character for Success
- Handling Finances
- Golden Rule Thinking
- Dating, Marriage, and Handling Peer Pressure
- Making Right Choices

A Must Read for Those Wanting a Bright Future!

For More Information Visit: www.AdvancePublishing.com/teens

What Others Say

"This book is filled with insights from a lifetime of experience by its author Carl Sommer. Not only does he draw from his own life as one who reached his wedding day as a virgin, but he gives hundreds of undeniable reasons why it is so much more important for today's sex-saturated society.

"Citing numerous authorities for the facts, he takes on the "safer sex" proponents and reveals the wide gaps in their arguments. Read why a counseling psychiatrist had to hide her identity when writing about this topic, and why Miss America had to fight the organizers to have her "abstinence" message approved as she started her reign.

"Young people are under even greater pressure from their peers and the prevailing culture to simply conform to the prevailing destructive forces with their misleading message that recreational sex has no downside. Parents, buy this book, read it for yourselves and pass it on to your kids. I can heartily recommend it and its approach to the important issue which it addresses."

Brian Cheyne, *Former Head of Department, Educational Guidance at Jeppe High School*

"I have just finished Sex-If You're Afraid of the Truth. I think this is a must read for every teenager, especially girls. Girls all too often don't realize that they hold the own key to their future. They give away their future far too easily."

Judy Hathcock, *High School Counselor*

"I really enjoyed reading the book and look forward to when it is published. I appreciate you writing on this topic. The message in your book is desperately needed in our society. The young people need to hear the truth that you write about."

Missy Patton, *Road Manager, Silver Ring Thing*

"This is a very needed book and well written. It is a quick and easy read. I especially like the stories; these will really speak to young people. I just hope it can be widely distributed. You obviously did a great deal of research and I like that you quote from many sources."

Barbara Horak, *Author and Speaker about Risks and Consequences of Premarital Sex*